MINOR SURGICAL PROCEDURES

POCKET GUIDE

DR. MOHAMED ELGENDY
LMCC, CCFP CANADA

DISCLAIMER

This pocket guide was developed with the assistance of advanced AI tools to streamline content generation. Every chapter has been thoroughly reviewed, edited, and authenticated by Dr. Mohamed Elgendy, LMCC, CCFP (Canada), ensuring accuracy, credibility, and clinical authenticity. The result is a modern, innovative reference that blends the efficiency of AI with the rigor of professional medical expertise.

This booklet summarizes common emergency and primary-care procedures using open-access guidance only; no proprietary or subscription content is reproduced. Procedural descriptions (steps, doses, device settings) are abbreviated for education and exam preparation and are not a step-by-step protocol or a substitute for clinical judgment.

Perform procedures only within your training and local scope, with appropriate consent, monitoring, equipment, and asepsis. Stop and escalate when red flags arise (e.g., airway compromise, uncontrolled bleeding, suspected deep-space infection, neurovascular injury) or when the situation exceeds your competence or resources.

Always verify current local guidelines, product monographs/labels, and institutional pathways; confirm patient-specific contraindications, allergies, and doses before use. Clinical responsibility remains with the treating clinician.

DEDICATION

This booklet is dedicated to the patients in rural and remote communities—whose resilience, trust, and courage guide every decision; to the clinicians, nurses, medics, and staff who deliver essential procedures with skill, compassion, and ingenuity despite distance and limited resources; to mentors and colleagues who share knowledge openly so care can remain safe and evidence-informed; and to my family, whose steady support makes this work possible. May this concise, open-access procedure booklet serve them all.

— Dr. Mohamed Elgendy

ABOUT THE AUTHIOR

Dr. Mohamed Elgendy is a licensed Canadian physician with the Licentiate of the Medical Council of Canada (LMCC) and Certification in Family Medicine (CCFP) from the College of Family Physicians of Canada.

He has extensive hands-on experience as both a rural emergency physician and family doctor, currently practicing in Saskatchewan, Canada. With a deep commitment to improving emergency and acute care in underserved communities, Dr. Elgendy focuses on practical, evidence-based emergency medicine adapted to the realities of rural practice.

His work bridges the gap between academic guidelines and frontline clinical realities, offering accessible, concise resources to help clinicians make confident, lifesaving decisions in resource-limited settings.

PROCEDURES INDEX — CATEGORIZED

MUSCULOSKELETAL & SOFT-TISSUE INJECTIONS/ ASPIRATIONS

SHOULDER JOINT STEROID INJECTION

INDICATIONS

1. Inflammatory joint conditions such as osteoarthritis, rheumatoid arthritis, adhesive capsulitis (frozen shoulder), and rotator cuff tendinopathy with associated bursitis.
2. Persistent pain and stiffness despite conservative management (analgesia, physiotherapy).
3. Diagnostic use to differentiate intra-articular from extra-articular pain sources.

CONTRAINDICATIONS

1. Absolute: overlying skin infection, suspected septic arthritis, uncontrolled coagulopathy, known allergy to steroid or anesthetic agents.
2. Relative: poorly controlled diabetes mellitus, repeated injections in same joint (>3–4/year), joint instability.

CONSENT

1. Explain purpose: reduce pain and inflammation, improve mobility.

2. Discuss benefits: symptom relief, improved function.
3. Discuss risks: infection, bleeding, allergic reaction, steroid flare, skin depigmentation, fat atrophy.
4. Discuss alternatives: physiotherapy, oral analgesia, observation, surgical referral.
5. Document verbal or written consent.

PREPARATION

1. Position: patient seated or supine, affected arm supported, shoulder relaxed.
2. Aseptic technique: sterile gloves, drapes, skin preparation with chlorhexidine or povidone-iodine.
3. Analgesia: local infiltration with 1% lidocaine or equivalent.
4. Ensure correct steroid selection and dose prepared.

EQUIPMENT

1. Sterile gloves, drapes, antiseptic solution.
2. Needle: 22G, 1.5 inches (adjust for patient size).
3. Syringes: 5 mL for injection.
4. Local anesthetic (1% lidocaine).
5. Injectable corticosteroid (e.g., triamcinolone acetonide 20–40 mg or methylprednisolone acetate 40 mg).
6. Sterile dressing.

PROCEDURE STEPS

1. Identify anatomical landmarks for approach: anterior (just lateral to coracoid process) or posterior (2 cm inferior and 1 cm medial to posterolateral acromion).
2. Prep skin with antiseptic and allow to dry completely.
3. Infiltrate skin and deeper tissues with local anesthetic.
4. Attach syringe containing steroid and anesthetic mixture to needle.
5. Insert needle into joint space using chosen approach; aspirate to ensure not in a blood vessel.
6. Inject contents slowly and steadily.
7. Withdraw needle, apply gentle pressure, and cover with sterile dressing.

COMPLICATIONS / SIDE EFFECTS

1. Post-injection steroid flare (increased pain for 24–48 hours).
2. Infection (septic arthritis).
3. Bleeding or hemarthrosis.
4. Allergic reaction.
5. Skin depigmentation or subcutaneous fat atrophy at injection site.
6. Transient hyperglycemia in diabetic patients.

AFTERCARE & MONITORING

1. Observe patient for immediate allergic reaction.
2. Advise rest of joint for 24–48 hours; avoid strenuous activity.
3. Monitor for infection signs: fever, redness, swelling, increasing pain.
4. Document procedure details and patient advice.

DISPOSITION

1. Discharge with follow-up in primary care or physiotherapy.
2. Urgent review if signs of infection develop.

REFERENCES

NHS – Shoulder Joint Injection. https://www.nhs.uk

HealthLink BC – Joint Injections. https://www.healthlinkbc.ca

Canadian Rheumatology Association – Patient Resources. https://rheum.ca

BC Guidelines – Musculoskeletal Injuries and Joint Injections. https://www2.gov.bc.ca

KNEE JOINT STEROID INJECTION

INDICATIONS

1. Symptomatic knee osteoarthritis with inflammatory flares or effusion.
2. Inflammatory arthropathies affecting the knee (e.g., rheumatoid arthritis, crystal arthropathy) after infection reasonably excluded.
3. Persistent pain and stiffness despite conservative care (activity modification, oral/topical analgesics, physiotherapy).
4. Diagnostic aid to distinguish intra-articular pain when combined with local anesthetic.

CONTRAINDICATIONS

1. Absolute: overlying skin/soft-tissue infection, suspected septic arthritis, true allergy to steroid or local anesthetic.
2. Relative: prosthetic knee (seek orthopedic input), uncontrolled coagulopathy or anticoagulation with additional bleeding risks, poorly controlled diabetes, recent fracture, planned surgery within weeks, repeated injections in same joint (>3–4/ year).

CONSENT

1. Purpose: reduce inflammation and pain, improve range of motion/function.
2. Benefits: short-term pain relief (often within 24–72 hours), improved mobility; may facilitate physiotherapy.
3. Risks: post-injection flare (24–48 h), infection, bleeding/hemarthrosis, skin depigmentation/fat atrophy, transient hyperglycemia, facial flushing, vasovagal reaction; rare chondrotoxicity with frequent injections.
4. Alternatives: oral/topical analgesics, physiotherapy, bracing, weight optimization, hyaluronic acid injection (if available), referral for surgical opinion.

PREPARATION

1. Position: patient supine with knee extended (or slight flexion with support); relax quadriceps.
2. Skin prep: chlorhexidine or povidone-iodine; full aseptic technique with sterile gloves and drape.
3. Analgesia: local infiltration with 1% lidocaine (or no-epi alternative).
4. If effusion present, plan to aspirate fully before steroid injection.

EQUIPMENT

1. Sterile gloves, drapes, antiseptic solution, sterile gauze.

2. Needle: typically 22G, 1.5 inch; consider 20–22G, 1.5–2 inch depending on body habitus/approach.

3. Syringes: 10–20 mL (aspiration) and 5 mL (injection).

4. Local anesthetic: 1% lidocaine (2–4 mL for anesthetic and to mix with steroid if desired).

5. Corticosteroid: triamcinolone acetonide 20–40 mg OR methylprednisolone acetate 40 mg (typical intra-articular dose).

6. Adhesive bandage/sterile dressing; specimen tubes if sending fluid.

PROCEDURE STEPS (LANDMARK – SUPEROLATERAL APPROACH)

1. Identify superolateral patellar border into the suprapatellar pouch with knee in extension.

2. Mark entry point ~1 cm superior and lateral to the patella; aim toward the intercondylar notch.

3. Skin antisepsis; allow to dry. Create small skin wheel of local anesthetic.

4. If effusion: attach 10–20 mL syringe to 20–22G needle, advance into joint; aspirate fluid completely. Send samples if indicated (cell count, Gram stain/culture, crystals).

5. Switch to injection syringe containing steroid ± small volume of local anesthetic. Aspirate to ensure not intravascular, then inject slowly without resistance.

6. Withdraw needle, apply gentle pressure, and place sterile dressing.

COMPLICATIONS / SIDE EFFECTS

1. Post-injection pain flare (self-limited).
2. Infection (septic arthritis) — educate on red flags and ensure follow-up.
3. Bleeding/hemarthrosis or bruise, vasovagal reaction.
4. Skin depigmentation and subcutaneous fat atrophy at injection site.
5. Transient hyperglycemia (diabetes; monitor and adjust therapy if needed).
6. Very rare: tendon or ligament injury if extra-articular injection; accelerated cartilage wear with frequent injections.

AFTERCARE & MONITORING

1. Observe briefly for vasovagal or allergic reactions.
2. Advise relative rest for 24–48 hours; ice as needed; avoid strenuous activity.
3. Warn about steroid flare; suggest simple analgesics if needed.
4. Diabetes: check glucose more frequently for 48–72 hours; expect transient elevations.
5. Return precautions: increasing pain, redness, warmth, fever, or inability to bear weight.

6. Document dose, agent, approach, lot numbers (if available), aspirate characteristics, and patient counseling.

DISPOSITION

1. Discharge with self-care instructions and physiotherapy plan as appropriate.
2. Arrange follow-up (e.g., 1–2 weeks) to assess response; avoid repeated injections more than every 3 months and limit to ≤3–4/year per joint.

REFERENCES

NHS — Steroid injections (general patient guidance). https://www.nhs.uk

NICE CKS — Intra-articular corticosteroid injections (open access). https://cks.nice.org.uk

HealthLink BC — Corticosteroid Injections. https://www.healthlinkbc.ca

Arthritis Society Canada — Joint injections overview. https://arthritis.ca

AAOS OrthoInfo — Cortisone Shot (open access patient info). https://orthoinfo.aaos.org

KNEE JOINT ASPIRATION

INDICATIONS

1. Diagnostic: suspected septic arthritis, crystal arthropathy (gout/pseudogout), unexplained effusion, hemarthrosis.
2. Therapeutic: relieve painful effusion, improve range of motion, facilitate subsequent intra-articular therapy.

CONTRAINDICATIONS

1. Absolute: overlying cellulitis/skin infection, true allergy to local anesthetic, non-correctable coagulopathy with high bleeding risk.
2. Relative: prosthetic knee (consult orthopedics), anticoagulation (weigh risks/benefits), recent joint replacement or planned surgery, severe joint destruction, uncooperative patient.

CONSENT

1. Purpose: remove fluid for analysis and/or relieve pain and stiffness.
2. Benefits: pain relief, improved mobility, diagnostic

clarity (cell count, culture, crystals).

3. Risks: infection, bleeding/hemarthrosis, pain, post-procedure swelling, vasovagal reaction, very rare injury to cartilage/ligament.

4. Alternatives: observation, analgesia, imaging, deferred aspiration after specialist review (if low suspicion for septic arthritis).

5. Document verbal/written consent and side (right/ left).

PREPARATION

1. Position: patient supine with knee in extension (or slight flexion supported by towel); relax quadriceps.

2. Asepsis: skin prep with chlorhexidine or povidone-iodine; sterile gloves and small drape.

3. Analgesia: local infiltration with 1% lidocaine; consider vapocoolant or topical anesthetic if needed.

4. If large effusion suspected, plan for complete aspiration before any injection.

EQUIPMENT

1. Sterile gloves, drapes, skin antiseptic, sterile gauze.

2. Needles: 20–22G (aspiration often easier with 18–20G if fluid is viscous); length 1.5–2 inches depending on habitus.

3. Syringes: 10–20 mL for aspiration; additional syringe if multiple draws expected.

4. Local anesthetic (1% lidocaine).

5. Specimen containers: sterile container for culture/ Gram stain; tube for cell count/differential; tube for crystal analysis per local lab protocol.

6. Adhesive bandage or sterile dressing; elastic wrap if compression desired.

PROCEDURE STEPS (LANDMARK – SUPEROLATERAL APPROACH)

1. Identify the superolateral patellar border and suprapatellar pouch with knee in extension.

2. Mark entry ~1 cm superior and lateral to the superolateral patella; aim toward the intercondylar notch.

3. Prep skin and allow antiseptic to dry; raise a skin wheal of local anesthetic and anesthetize the tract.

4. Attach a 10–20 mL syringe to a 20G needle (or 18–20G if fluid is thick). Advance into the joint while applying gentle negative pressure.

5. Once fluid returns, aspirate as much as possible. If needed, pause and switch to a fresh syringe without moving needle tip.

6. Collect samples as indicated: cell count/ differential, Gram stain and culture, and crystals (follow lab handling requirements).

7. Withdraw needle, apply pressure, and place a sterile dressing; optional light compression wrap.

COMPLICATIONS / SIDE EFFECTS

1. Post-procedure discomfort or transient swelling.
2. Hemarthrosis or bruising (higher risk with anticoagulation/coagulopathy).
3. Infection (iatrogenic septic arthritis) — rare but serious.
4. Vasovagal syncope.
5. Very rare: injury to cartilage, tendon or ligament; synovial fluid leak/persistent drainage.

AFTERCARE & MONITORING

1. Observe briefly for vasovagal reaction; reassess pain and mobility.
2. Relative rest and ice for 24–48 hours; consider compression wrap.
3. Educate on red flags: increasing pain, redness, warmth, fever, inability to bear weight.
4. If crystals or infection suspected, arrange appropriate follow-up and treatment; document volume/appearance of fluid and tests sent.

DISPOSITION

1. Discharge with self-care instructions if stable and infection unlikely.

2. Urgent specialist consultation/admission if septic arthritis suspected or patient systemically unwell.

REFERENCES

NICE CKS — Intra-articular corticosteroid injections: general safety and technique (open access). https://cks.nice.org.uk

NHS — Steroid injections and joint procedures (patient info). https://www.nhs.uk

HealthLink BC — Joint injections and aftercare (patient info). https://www.healthlinkbc.ca

Arthritis Society Canada — Joint injections and aspirations overview. https://arthritis.ca

AAOS OrthoInfo — Joint procedures and aftercare (patient info). https://orthoinfo.aaos.org

OLECRANON BURSITIS – ASPIRATION ± STEROID INJECTION

INDICATIONS

1. Diagnostic: rule out septic bursitis or crystal disease (gout/pseudogout).
2. Therapeutic: relieve tense, painful swelling; recurrent aseptic bursitis after failed conservative care.
3. Consider steroid injection ONLY after infection is reasonably excluded.

CONTRAINDICATIONS

1. Absolute: overlying cellulitis, suspected septic bursitis without ability to send cultures, true allergy to agents.
2. Relative: anticoagulation/coagulopathy, poorly controlled diabetes (for steroid), recurrent trauma/pressure, prosthetic material nearby.

CONSENT

1. Purpose: remove fluid for diagnosis/symptom relief; optional steroid to reduce recurrence.
2. Benefits: pain relief, faster functional recovery, diagnostic clarity.
3. Risks: infection, bleeding/hematoma, post-procedure pain, skin atrophy/depigmentation (with steroid), recurrence.
4. Alternatives: rest/ice/compression/NSAIDs, padding, activity modification, aspiration without steroid, referral.

PREPARATION

1. Position: patient seated or supine with elbow flexed ~45–90°, forearm supported.
2. Asepsis: chlorhexidine or povidone-iodine; sterile gloves/drape.
3. Analgesia: local infiltration with 1% lidocaine; consider vapocoolant/topical first.

EQUIPMENT

1. Sterile gloves, small sterile drape, antiseptic, gauze.
2. Needles: 18–22G (larger if fluid viscous); length 1–1.5 in.
3. Syringes: 10–20 mL for aspiration; 3–5 mL if injecting.
4. Local anesthetic (1% lidocaine).

5. Specimen containers: culture/Gram stain, cell count/diff, crystals (per lab protocol).

6. Elastic/compression wrap; protective elbow padding.

PROCEDURE STEPS – ASPIRATION

1. Identify the most fluctuant point over the olecranon; avoid medial approach (ulnar nerve).

2. Prep and anesthetize skin/tract. Enter bursa with 18–22G needle perpendicular or slightly oblique.

3. Apply gentle suction; aspirate completely if possible. If thick, consider larger needle.

4. Send fluid as indicated: Gram stain/culture, cell count/differential, crystals.

5. Withdraw needle, apply firm pressure, place sterile dressing, then compression wrap.

OPTIONAL – STEROID INJECTION (ONLY IF ASEPTIC)

1. Confirm no clinical concern for infection; ideally review preliminary microscopy if available.

2. Inject small dose into bursal space: triamcinolone acetonide 10–20 mg OR methylprednisolone acetate 20 mg, often mixed with 1–2 mL lidocaine.

3. Inject slowly; avoid skin infiltration with steroid to reduce atrophy/depigmentation.

COMPLICATIONS / SIDE EFFECTS

1. Infection (iatrogenic septic bursitis), bleeding/ hematoma, pain flare.
2. Skin atrophy/depigmentation (steroid), sinus tract/ persistent drainage, recurrence.
3. Vasovagal syncope; rare injury to ulnar nerve (avoid medial entry).

AFTERCARE & MONITORING

1. Compression wrap for 24–48 h; ice/elevation; avoid pressure on elbow; use padding.
2. Analgesia: acetaminophen/NSAIDs if appropriate.
3. Return precautions: redness, warmth, fever, increasing pain/drainage.
4. If crystals or infection suspected/confirmed: arrange treatment and follow-up; document volume/appearance and tests sent.

DISPOSITION

1. Discharge with self-care, padding, and activity modification if stable.
2. Urgent review/admission if systemic illness or septic bursitis suspected.

REFERENCES

NHS — Bursitis (patient guidance). https://www.nhs.uk

MyHealth.Alberta.ca — Bursitis care and procedures. https://myhealth.alberta.ca

HealthLinkBC — Bursitis:careandself-management. https://www.healthlinkbc.ca

Arthritis Society Canada — Bursitis overview. https://arthritis.ca

AAOS OrthoInfo — Elbow (Olecranon) Bursitis: patient information. https://orthoinfo.aaos.org

PREPATELLAR BURSITIS – ASPIRATION ± STEROID INJECTION

INDICATIONS

1. Diagnostic: rule out septic bursitis or crystal disease (gout/pseudogout) in an anterior knee swelling.
2. Therapeutic: relieve tense, painful prepatellar swelling; recurrent aseptic bursitis after failed conservative care.
3. Steroid injection ONLY when infection is reasonably excluded.

CONTRAINDICATIONS

1. Absolute: overlying cellulitis/skin infection, suspected septic bursitis if cultures cannot be sent, true allergy to agents.
2. Relative: anticoagulation/coagulopathy, poorly controlled diabetes (for steroid), recurrent kneeling/pressure without ability to modify, open wounds or abrasions over bursa.

CONSENT

1. Purpose: remove fluid for diagnosis/symptom relief; optional steroid to reduce inflammation/ recurrence.
2. Benefits: pain relief, improved function, diagnostic clarity.
3. Risks: infection, bleeding/hematoma, post-procedure pain, skin atrophy/depigmentation (with steroid), recurrence, sinus tract/persistent drainage.
4. Alternatives: rest/ice/compression/NSAIDs, knee padding, activity modification, aspiration without steroid, referral.

PREPARATION

1. Position: patient supine or seated with knee slightly flexed (rolled towel under knee) to relax anterior soft tissues.
2. Asepsis: skin prep with chlorhexidine or povidone-iodine; sterile gloves and small drape.
3. Analgesia: local infiltration with 1% lidocaine; consider topical/vapocoolant first.

EQUIPMENT

1. Sterile gloves, small sterile drape, antiseptic swabs, gauze, adhesive bandage.
2. Needles: 18–22G (larger if viscous fluid); length 1–1.5 in.

3. Syringes: 10–20 mL for aspiration; 3–5 mL if injecting.
4. Local anesthetic (1% lidocaine).
5. Specimen containers: culture/Gram stain, cell count/differential, crystals (per lab protocol).
6. Elastic/compression wrap; protective knee padding.

PROCEDURE STEPS – ASPIRATION

1. Identify the most fluctuant point directly over the prepatellar bursa (anterior to patella); mark entry site.
2. Prep and anesthetize skin/tract. Enter bursa perpendicular or slightly oblique to the skin to minimize persistent leakage.
3. Apply gentle suction and aspirate completely if possible. If fluid is thick, consider a larger bore needle (18–20G).
4. Collect specimens as indicated: Gram stain/ culture, cell count/differential, and crystals (follow lab handling requirements).
5. Withdraw needle, apply firm pressure, place sterile dressing, then a snug compression wrap to reduce re-accumulation.

OPTIONAL – STEROID INJECTION (ONLY IF ASEPTIC)

1. Proceed only when there is no clinical concern for

infection; ideally review preliminary microscopy if available.

2. Inject small dose into the bursal space: triamcinolone acetonide 10–20 mg OR methylprednisolone acetate 20 mg, often mixed with 1–2 mL of 1% lidocaine.

3. Inject slowly; avoid intradermal steroid deposition to reduce risk of skin atrophy/depigmentation.

COMPLICATIONS / SIDE EFFECTS

1. Infection (iatrogenic septic bursitis), bleeding/ hematoma, pain flare.

2. Skin atrophy/depigmentation with steroid, sinus tract/persistent drainage, recurrence (especially with ongoing kneeling/pressure).

3. Vasovagal syncope; rare injury to nearby cutaneous nerves.

AFTERCARE & MONITORING

1. Compression wrap for 24–48 h; ice and elevation; avoid kneeling or direct pressure; use protective padding.

2. Analgesia: acetaminophen/NSAIDs if appropriate.

3. Return precautions: increasing pain, redness, warmth, fever, or draining sinus.

4. If crystals or infection suspected/confirmed: arrange treatment and follow-up; document volume/appearance and tests sent.

DISPOSITION

1. Discharge with self-care, padding, and activity modification if stable.
2. Urgent review/admission if systemic illness or septic bursitis suspected.

REFERENCES

NHS — Bursitis (patient guidance). https://www.nhs.uk

MyHealth.Alberta.ca — Bursitis care and procedures. https://myhealth.alberta.ca

HealthLink BC — Bursitis: care and self-management. https://www.healthlinkbc.ca

Arthritis Society Canada — Bursitis overview. https://arthritis.ca

AAOS OrthoInfo — Knee Bursitis (Prepatellar): patient information. https://orthoinfo.aaos.org

GREATER TROCHANTERIC PAIN SYNDROME (TROCHANTERIC BURSITIS) – STEROID INJECTION

INDICATIONS

1. Lateral hip pain/tenderness over the greater trochanter with sleep disturbance (lying on side) and pain on single-leg stance or resisted abduction.
2. Failure of conservative care (activity modification, NSAIDs/topicals, physiotherapy focusing on hip abductor/IT band).
3. Diagnostic–therapeutic trial to confirm peritrochanteric inflammation as pain source.

CONTRAINDICATIONS

1. Overlying skin infection or suspected deep infection.
2. True allergy to corticosteroid or local anesthetic.
3. Relative: poorly controlled diabetes (transient hyperglycemia), anticoagulation/coagulopathy, prior multiple injections, suspected gluteal tendon

tear (consider imaging/specialist).

CONSENT

1. Purpose: reduce peritrochanteric inflammation/ pain and improve function.
2. Benefits: short-term pain relief (often within 24–72 h), improved sleep/function; may facilitate rehab.
3. Risks: pain flare, bleeding/bruising, infection, skin depigmentation/fat atrophy, transient paresthesia (nearby cutaneous nerves), very rare tendon injury if intratendinous, transient hyperglycemia.
4. Alternatives: physiotherapy (hip abductor strengthening, ITB stretching), oral/topical analgesics, activity modification, shockwave therapy, referral if refractory.

PREPARATION

1. Position: lateral decubitus with affected side up (or supine); slight internal rotation of leg to expose lateral trochanter.
2. Landmark: palpate the point of maximal tenderness along the posterolateral facet of the greater trochanter.
3. Asepsis: prep with chlorhexidine or povidone-iodine; sterile gloves; small sterile drape.
4. Local anesthesia: small intradermal wheel and tract with 1% lidocaine.

EQUIPMENT

1. Sterile gloves, antiseptic swabs, gauze, small sterile drape, adhesive bandage.
2. Needle: 22–25G, length 1.5–3.5 inches depending on body habitus.
3. Syringe: 3–5 mL.
4. Injectate (typical): triamcinolone acetonide 20–40 mg OR methylprednisolone acetate 40 mg, often mixed with 1–3 mL of 1% lidocaine (no epinephrine).

PROCEDURE STEPS – LANDMARK PERITROCHANTERIC INJECTION

1. Mark the most tender point over the greater trochanter.
2. Insert the needle perpendicular to skin toward bone until bony contact with the trochanter is felt; withdraw 2–3 mm to position in the bursal/ peritendinous plane (avoid intratendinous injection).
3. Aspirate to ensure not intravascular; inject slowly 1–3 mL with minimal resistance. Use a gentle 'fan' technique to distribute around the tender area.
4. Withdraw needle, apply pressure, and place a small dressing.

COMPLICATIONS / SIDE EFFECTS

1. Pain flare (24–48 h), bruising, local skin changes (atrophy/depigmentation).
2. Infection (rare), transient numbness, very rare tendon injury if intratendinous or with repeated injections.
3. Transient hyperglycemia (monitor in diabetes for 48–72 h).

AFTERCARE & MONITORING

1. Relative rest for 24–48 h; ice as needed; avoid prolonged side-lying on the affected side.
2. Begin/continue physiotherapy after pain settles (3–7 days): hip abductor strengthening and IT band stretching.
3. Warn about red flags: increasing pain, redness, warmth, fever, progressive weakness.
4. Plan review in 1–2 weeks; avoid frequent repeat injections (generally ≥3 months apart; limit to ≤3–4/year).

DISPOSITION

1. Discharge with instructions and follow-up. Consider imaging/referral if poor response or suspected gluteal tendinopathy/tear.

REFERENCES

NHS — Hip (trochanteric) bursitis: patient guidance. https://www.nhs.uk

HealthLink BC — Hip bursitis: overview and self-care. https://www.healthlinkbc.ca

MyHealth.Alberta.ca — Hip bursitis care instructions. https://myhealth.alberta.ca

Arthritis Society Canada — Bursitis overview & hip pain resources. https://arthritis.ca

NICE CKS — Hip pain in adults (includes greater trochanteric pain syndrome). https://cks.nice.org.uk

AAOS OrthoInfo — Hip Bursitis (Trochanteric): patient information. https://orthoinfo.aaos.org

DE QUERVAIN'S TENOSYNOVITIS (FIRST DORSAL COMPARTMENT) – STEROID INJECTION

INDICATIONS

1. Painful radial wrist with APL/EPB tendon sheath tenderness, positive Finkelstein/Eichhoff tests.
2. Failure of conservative care (activity modification, thumb-spica splint, NSAIDs/analgesics) or significant functional impairment.
3. Diagnostic–therapeutic trial to confirm tendon-sheath inflammation as the pain source.

CONTRAINDICATIONS

1. Overlying skin infection or suspected tendon-sheath infection.
2. True allergy to corticosteroid or local anesthetic.
3. Relative: poorly controlled diabetes (transient hyperglycemia risk), anticoagulation/coagulopathy, prior multiple injections to the same site.

CONSENT

1. Purpose: reduce pain and swelling within the APL/EPB tendon sheath and improve function.

2. Benefits: high short-term success for many patients; may avoid surgery.

3. Risks: pain flare (24–48 h), bleeding/bruising, infection, skin depigmentation/fat atrophy, transient numbness (superficial radial nerve irritation), very rare tendon rupture, transient hyperglycemia.

4. Alternatives: splinting, activity modification, oral/topical analgesics, hand therapy, surgical release if refractory.

PREPARATION

1. Identify maximal tenderness over the radial styloid (first dorsal compartment).

2. Position: forearm supported, wrist slightly ulnar-deviated; hand supinated.

3. Asepsis: chlorhexidine or povidone-iodine; sterile gloves; small sterile drape.

4. Local anesthesia: small intradermal wheel of 1% lidocaine if desired.

EQUIPMENT

1. Sterile gloves, antiseptic swabs, gauze, small sterile drape, adhesive bandage.

2. Needle: 25–27G, ½–1 inch; Syringe: 1–3 mL.

3. Injectate (typical): triamcinolone acetonide 10 mg OR methylprednisolone acetate 20 mg, often mixed with 0.5–1 mL of 1% lidocaine.

PROCEDURE STEPS – LANDMARK INJECTION

1. Palpate the first dorsal compartment (APL/EPB) just proximal to the radial styloid; mark the most tender point.
2. Insert needle at ~30–45° along the tendon sheath, parallel to the tendons; avoid intratendinous injection.
3. Advance gently; a subtle 'give' may be felt entering the sheath. Aspirate to ensure not intravascular.
4. Inject 0.5–1.0 mL slowly. If marked resistance or tendon pain, withdraw slightly and reposition in the sheath.
5. Withdraw needle, apply gentle pressure, and place a small dressing. Consider a short course of thumb-spica splinting.

COMPLICATIONS / SIDE EFFECTS

1. Pain flare, bruising, local skin atrophy/ depigmentation, fat atrophy.
2. Superficial radial nerve irritation (paresthesia), infection (rare), bleeding/hematoma.
3. Very rare: tendon rupture; risk increases with

repeated injections.

4. Transient hyperglycemia; counsel patients with diabetes to monitor closely for 48–72 h.

AFTERCARE & MONITORING

1. Rest wrist/thumb for 24–48 h; avoid repetitive grasping or ulnar deviation; ice as needed.

2. Warn about red flags: increasing pain, redness, warmth, fever, progressive numbness.

3. Consider splinting and hand therapy for rehabilitation.

4. If persistent or recurrent symptoms after 1–2 injections spaced ≥6–8 weeks, consider referral for surgical release.

DISPOSITION

1. Discharge with instructions and follow-up in 1–2 weeks to assess response.

REFERENCES

NHS — De Quervain's tenosynovitis (patient guidance). https://www.nhs.uk

MyHealth.Alberta.ca — De Quervain's tenosynovitis: care instructions. https://myhealth.alberta.ca

HealthLink BC — De Quervain's disease: overview and self-care. https://www.healthlinkbc.ca

AAOS OrthoInfo — De Quervain's Tendinosis (patient information). https://orthoinfo.aaos.org

British Society for Surgery of the Hand (BSSH) — Patient leaflet: De Quervain's. https://www.bssh.ac.uk

TRIGGER FINGER (FLEXOR TENDON SHEATH) – STEROID INJECTION

INDICATIONS

1. Painful locking/catching of a finger or thumb with palpable A1 pulley tenderness.
2. Failure of conservative therapy (activity modification, splinting, NSAIDs) or significant functional impairment.
3. Diagnostic-therapeutic trial to confirm tendon sheath inflammation as pain source.

CONTRAINDICATIONS

1. Overlying skin infection or suspected flexor tendon sheath infection.
2. True allergy to local anesthetic or corticosteroid.
3. Relative: poorly controlled diabetes (risk of transient hyperglycemia), anticoagulation/ coagulopathy, prior multiple injections in the same digit.

CONSENT

1. Purpose: reduce pain, catching/locking, and

improve function.

2. Benefits: high short-term success in many patients; may avoid surgery.

3. Risks: pain flare (24–48 h), bleeding/bruising, infection, skin depigmentation or fat atrophy at puncture site, tendon rupture (rare), transient hyperglycemia, digital nerve irritation.

4. Alternatives: rest/splinting, NSAIDs/topicals, hand therapy, or surgical A1 pulley release if refractory.

PREPARATION

1. Identify affected digit; palpate A1 pulley at the level of the MCP joint (volar surface).

2. Position hand supine with wrist slightly extended; support on a sterile field.

3. Skin prep with chlorhexidine or povidone-iodine; sterile gloves; optional sterile fenestrated drape.

4. Local anesthesia: small intradermal wheel of 1% lidocaine if desired.

EQUIPMENT

1. Sterile gloves, antiseptic swabs, small sterile drape, gauze, adhesive bandage.

2. Needle: 25–27G, ½–1 inch; Syringe: 1–3 mL.

3. Injectate (typical): triamcinolone acetonide 10 mg OR methylprednisolone acetate 20 mg, often mixed with 0.5–1 mL of 1% lidocaine.

PROCEDURE STEPS – A1 PULLEY SHEATH INJECTION

1. Palpate the A1 pulley (over the MCP joint crease). Mark the most tender nodule.

2. Enter at the midline of the volar finger/thumb just proximal to the MCP crease. Aim distally at ~30–45° along the tendon sheath.

3. Advance needle; a subtle "give" may be felt on entering the sheath. Avoid injecting directly into the tendon substance.

4. Aspirate to ensure not intravascular. Inject slowly 0.5–1.0 mL. If marked resistance or tendon pain, withdraw slightly and reposition.

5. Apply gentle pressure, then a small adhesive bandage. Consider short-term splinting for comfort.

COMPLICATIONS / SIDE EFFECTS

1. Pain flare, bruising, local skin changes (depigmentation, atrophy).

2. Infection, digital nerve irritation, rare tendon rupture (risk increases with repeated injections).

3. Transient hyperglycemia; counsel patients with diabetes to monitor.

AFTERCARE & MONITORING

1. Rest the hand and avoid forceful gripping for 24–48 hours; ice prn.

2. Warn about red flags: increasing pain, redness, warmth, fever, numbness.

3. Diabetes: check glucose more frequently for 48–72 hours.

4. If symptoms persist or recur after 1–2 injections separated by ≥6–8 weeks, consider surgical referral.

DISPOSITION

1. Discharge with instructions and follow-up (1–2 weeks) to assess response.

REFERENCES

NHS — Trigger finger (patient guidance). https://www.nhs.uk

MyHealth.Alberta.ca — Trigger finger overview and care. https://myhealth.alberta.ca

HealthLink BC — Trigger finger information. https://www.healthlinkbc.ca

AAOS OrthoInfo — Trigger Finger: patient information. https://orthoinfo.aaos.org

British Society for Surgery of the Hand (BSSH) — Patient leaflet: Trigger finger. https://www.bssh.ac.uk

LATERAL EPICONDYLITIS (TENNIS ELBOW) – STEROID INJECTION

INDICATIONS

1. Persistent lateral elbow pain with tenderness over the common extensor origin (ECRB), grip-related pain, and failed conservative care (rest, activity modification, brace, physiotherapy, NSAIDs).
2. Significant functional impairment affecting work/ADLs.
3. Diagnostic–therapeutic trial to confirm peritendinous inflammation as pain source.

CONTRAINDICATIONS

1. Overlying skin infection or suspected deep infection.
2. True allergy to corticosteroid or local anesthetic.
3. Relative: poorly controlled diabetes (transient hyperglycemia), anticoagulation/coagulopathy, prior multiple injections at the same site, suspected tendon tear.

CONSENT

1. Purpose: reduce pain and inflammation at the common extensor origin and improve function.

2. Benefits: short-term pain relief (often within 24–72 h) and improved function; may facilitate rehab.

3. Risks: pain flare, bleeding/bruising, infection, skin depigmentation or fat atrophy (if superficial), transient radial nerve irritation, very rare tendon weakening/rupture (avoid intratendinous injection), transient hyperglycemia.

4. Alternatives: continued conservative therapy (brace, eccentric strengthening), physiotherapy, topical/oral analgesics, shockwave therapy, referral for surgical evaluation if refractory.

PREPARATION

1. Identify maximal tenderness 1–2 cm distal/ anterior to the lateral epicondyle (common extensor origin).

2. Position: patient seated; elbow flexed ~90°, forearm pronated, wrist slightly flexed to relax extensors.

3. Asepsis: skin prep with chlorhexidine or povidone-iodine; sterile gloves; small sterile drape.

4. Optional: mark superficial vessels to avoid; consider ultrasound if anatomy uncertain.

EQUIPMENT

1. Sterile gloves, antiseptic swabs, gauze, small sterile drape, adhesive bandage.
2. Needle: 25–27G, 1 inch; Syringe: 1–3 mL.
3. Injectate (typical): triamcinolone acetonide 10–20 mg OR methylprednisolone acetate 20–40 mg, often mixed with 0.5–1 mL of 1% lidocaine (no epinephrine).

PROCEDURE STEPS – LANDMARK PERITENDINOUS INJECTION

1. Palpate and mark the point of maximal tenderness at the common extensor origin.
2. Insert needle perpendicular to skin toward the tendon origin until firm resistance is felt; withdraw 1–2 mm to avoid intratendinous placement.
3. Aspirate to ensure not intravascular; inject a small test amount to confirm minimal resistance and patient comfort.
4. Use a 'peppering' technique: distribute 0.5–1.0 mL in 3–4 directions around the tendon origin (peritendinous plane), avoiding direct intratendinous injection.
5. Withdraw needle, apply pressure for hemostasis, and place a small dressing. Consider forearm strap/brace after injection.

COMPLICATIONS / SIDE EFFECTS

1. Pain flare (24–48 h), bruising, local skin changes (atrophy/depigmentation).
2. Infection (rare), transient radial nerve irritation/ paresthesia.
3. Very rare: tendon weakening/rupture with intratendinous steroid or repeated injections.
4. Transient hyperglycemia (monitor in diabetes for 48–72 h).

AFTERCARE & MONITORING

1. Relative rest for 24–48 h; ice as needed; avoid heavy gripping or resisted wrist extension.
2. Begin/continue physiotherapy focusing on eccentric wrist extensor strengthening after pain settles (typically 3–7 days).
3. Warn about red flags: increasing pain, redness, warmth, fever, progressive numbness/weakness.
4. Plan review in 1–2 weeks; avoid frequent repeat injections (generally ≥3 months between injections, limit total number).

DISPOSITION

1. Discharge with instructions and follow-up. Consider workplace/ergonomic modifications and bracing.

REFERENCES

NHS — Tennis elbow (patient guidance). https://www.nhs.uk

HealthLink BC — Tennis elbow: overview and self-care. https://www.healthlinkbc.ca

MyHealth.Alberta.ca — Tennis elbow care instructions. https://myhealth.alberta.ca

AAOS OrthoInfo — Tennis Elbow (Lateral Epicondylitis): patient information. https://orthoinfo.aaos.org

NICE CKS — Corticosteroid injections: general safety considerations (open access). https://cks.nice.org.uk

CARPAL TUNNEL SYNDROME – STEROID INJECTION

INDICATIONS

1. Paresthesia, pain, or nocturnal symptoms in median nerve distribution with clinical CTS diagnosis.
2. Failure of conservative care (night wrist splint, activity modification, NSAIDs/topicals) or need for short-term relief while awaiting definitive management.
3. Diagnostic–therapeutic trial to assess response and confirm CTS as symptom source.

CONTRAINDICATIONS

1. Overlying skin infection at injection site or suspected deep space infection.
2. True allergy to corticosteroid or local anesthetic.
3. Relative: poorly controlled diabetes (transient hyperglycemia risk), anticoagulation/coagulopathy, prior multiple injections with diminishing benefit, severe thenar atrophy or

profound motor deficit (consider urgent surgical evaluation).

CONSENT

1. Purpose: reduce median nerve/tendon sheath inflammation to relieve pain and paresthesia.
2. Benefits: short-term symptom improvement; may delay/avoid surgery in some cases.
3. Risks: pain flare, bleeding/bruising, infection, skin depigmentation/fat atrophy, transient numbness, median nerve irritation or injury (rare), tendon injury (rare), transient hyperglycemia.
4. Alternatives: wrist splinting (especially at night), activity modification/ergonomics, oral/ topical analgesics, hand therapy, definitive surgical decompression for persistent or severe cases.

PREPARATION

1. Identify palmaris longus (PL) tendon by opposing thumb and little finger with wrist flexion; if absent, use flexor carpi radialis (FCR) as landmark.
2. Position: patient seated; forearm supinated; wrist slightly extended on a towel roll; fingers relaxed.
3. Asepsis: skin prep with chlorhexidine or povidone-iodine; sterile gloves; small sterile drape.
4. Local anesthesia: small intradermal wheel of 1% lidocaine if desired (avoid epinephrine).

EQUIPMENT

1. Sterile gloves, antiseptic swabs, gauze, small sterile drape, adhesive bandage.
2. Needle: 25–27G, 1–1.5 inch; Syringe: 1–3 mL.
3. Injectate (typical): triamcinolone acetonide 10–20 mg OR methylprednisolone acetate 20–40 mg, usually mixed with 0.5–1 mL of 1% lidocaine (no epinephrine).

PROCEDURE STEPS – LANDMARK INJECTION (ULNAR TO PL)

1. Palpate the distal wrist crease. Identify the PL tendon (or FCR if PL absent).
2. Mark an entry point just ulnar to the PL tendon at or slightly proximal to the distal wrist crease, avoiding the radial artery (radial side) and ulnar neurovascular bundle (ulnar side).
3. Insert the needle at ~30–45° distally, parallel to the flexor tendons, advancing 1–2 cm into the carpal tunnel. **Do not inject if the patient reports paresthesia or electric-shock pain**—withdraw slightly and redirect.
4. Aspirate to ensure not intravascular; then inject 0.5–1.0 mL slowly with minimal resistance.
5. Withdraw the needle, apply gentle pressure, and place a small dressing. Consider short-term neutral-position wrist splinting.

COMPLICATIONS / SIDE EFFECTS

1. Pain flare (24–48 h), bruising, local skin changes (atrophy/depigmentation).
2. Infection (rare), transient median nerve irritation/ neuritis, hematoma.
3. Very rare: intraneural injection or tendon injury; prevent by avoiding injection when paresthesia occurs and by correct needle path.
4. Transient hyperglycemia (monitor in diabetes for 48–72 h).

AFTERCARE & MONITORING

1. Relative rest for 24–48 h; avoid forceful gripping or repetitive wrist flexion/extension; ice as needed.
2. Night splinting for symptom control; consider hand therapy and ergonomic modifications.
3. Warn about red flags: increasing pain, redness, warmth, fever, progressive numbness/weakness or thenar weakness.
4. Follow-up in 1–2 weeks to assess response. Limit repeat injections (generally ≥3 months between injections; total number should be limited).

DISPOSITION

1. Discharge with instructions and follow-up. Refer for surgical evaluation if severe symptoms, motor deficit, or poor response to injection/conservative therapy.

REFERENCES

NHS — Carpal tunnel syndrome (patient guidance). https://www.nhs.uk

NICE CKS — Carpal tunnel syndrome (open access). https://cks.nice.org.uk

HealthLink BC — Carpal tunnel syndrome: overview and self-care. https://www.healthlinkbc.ca

MyHealth.Alberta.ca — Carpal tunnel syndrome care instructions. https://myhealth.alberta.ca

AAOS OrthoInfo — Carpal Tunnel Syndrome (patient information). https://orthoinfo.aaos.org

British Society for Surgery of the Hand (BSSH) — Patient leaflet: Carpal tunnel syndrome. https://www.bssh.ac.uk

GANGLION CYST ASPIRATION

INDICATIONS

1. Symptomatic dorsal wrist ganglion (pain, reduced range/grip, cosmetic concern).
2. Mucous (digital) cyst at DIP joint with discomfort or nail deformity.
3. Diagnostic confirmation when cystic lesion vs. solid mass uncertain after exam/ultrasound.

CONTRAINDICATIONS

1. Overlying cellulitis/skin infection or open wounds.
2. Suspected solid tumor or vascular lesion; atypical mass features.
3. Relative: volar wrist ganglion close to radial artery/median nerve (consider surgical/US-guided approach), anticoagulation/coagulopathy.

CONSENT

1. Purpose: remove gelatinous fluid to relieve symptoms and confirm diagnosis; recurrence risk discussed.

2. Benefits: symptom relief, minimal invasiveness.

3. Risks: recurrence (common), pain flare, bleeding/ hematoma, infection, skin depigmentation/ fat atrophy (if steroid used), nerve/artery injury (especially volar wrist), tendon irritation.

4. Alternatives: observation, splinting/activity modification, surgical excision if persistent or recurrent.

PREPARATION

1. Confirm cyst location and relation to critical structures (clinical exam ± ultrasound if uncertain).

2. Position: hand/wrist well supported; expose and mark most fluctuant point.

3. Asepsis: chlorhexidine or povidone–iodine; sterile gloves; small drape.

4. Local anesthesia: small intradermal wheel and tract with 1% lidocaine.

EQUIPMENT

1. Sterile gloves, antiseptic swabs, gauze, small sterile drape, adhesive bandage.

2. Needle: 18–22G (larger bore helps with viscous fluid); length 1–1.5 in.

3. Syringe: 5–10 mL for aspiration; second syringe if needed.

4. Optional injectate (aseptic cases only): small

volume of corticosteroid (e.g., triamcinolone acetonide 10 mg) to reduce short-term recurrence; discuss risks and variable evidence.

5. Elastic/compression wrap or firm dressing.

PROCEDURE STEPS – DORSAL WRIST (LANDMARK ASPIRATION)

1. Identify the cyst dome; avoid crossing extensor tendons directly if possible.

2. Prep and anesthetize skin/tract. Enter cyst perpendicular or slightly oblique; advance until cavity is reached (loss of resistance).

3. Apply steady suction; aspirate gelatinous fluid completely. Gentle 'fenestration' with a few passes may help collapse the cavity (avoid excessive trauma).

4. If opting for steroid in aseptic cases, inject a small amount after full aspiration; do NOT inject if any suspicion of infection.

5. Withdraw needle, apply firm pressure, and place compression dressing to reduce re-accumulation.

DIGITAL MUCOUS CYST (DIP) – NOTES

1. Approach dorsally just proximal to the nail fold; avoid nail matrix and extensor tendon.

2. Aspiration only; if considering steroid, use minimal dose and avoid intradermal injection to

reduce skin atrophy/ulceration risk.

3. High recurrence; consider hand surgery referral for persistent or recurrent cases.

COMPLICATIONS / SIDE EFFECTS

1. Recurrence (common, especially wrist and mucous cysts).

2. Pain flare, bruising/hematoma, infection.

3. Skin atrophy/depigmentation (steroid), tendon irritation/rupture (rare).

4. Neurovascular injury risk higher with volar wrist lesions (radial artery, palmar cutaneous branch of median nerve).

AFTERCARE & MONITORING

1. Compression for 24–48 h; relative rest; avoid repetitive strain for several days.

2. Ice/analgesics as needed. Educate on signs of infection or neurovascular compromise.

3. If recurrence or persistent symptoms, discuss surgical options; document size, site, volume aspirated, and any injectate.

DISPOSITION

1. Discharge with instructions and follow-up in 1–2 weeks. Earlier review if pain, redness, numbness, or rapid re-accumulation.

REFERENCES

NHS — Ganglion cyst (patient guidance). https://www.nhs.uk

MyHealth.Alberta.ca — Ganglion cyst: care instructions. https://myhealth.alberta.ca

HealthLink BC — Ganglion cysts: overview and self-care. https://www.healthlinkbc.ca

AAOS OrthoInfo — Ganglion Cyst of the Wrist and Hand (patient information). https://orthoinfo.aaos.org

British Society for Surgery of the Hand (BSSH) — Patient leaflet: Ganglion cysts. https://www.bssh.ac.uk

DERMATOLOGY –
PROCEDURES & LESION CARE

RURAL PROCEDURES POCKET GUIDE
— CONTENTS (CATEGORIZED)

MUSCULOSKELETAL & SOFT-TISSUE INJECTIONS/ASPIRATIONS

ENT / EYE

1. Anterior nasal packing for epistaxis
2. Peritonsillar abscess — needle aspiration
3. Ear canal irrigation & cerumen removal
4. Removal of foreign bodies — eye/ear/nose (and skin/soft tissue)

GENERAL SURGICAL/ED INFECTIONS

1. Cutaneous abscess — I&D
2. Pilonidal abscess — I&D

GU & WOMEN'S HEALTH

1. Bladder catheterization — urethral (male & female)
2. Bartholin gland abscess — I&D with Word catheter
3. Pap test — cervical cytology (collection)

(All topics above are prepared as ≤2-page, open-access guides.)

SKIN BIOPSY —
SHAVE & PUNCH TECHNIQUES

INDICATIONS

1. Diagnosis of suspicious lesions (neoplastic, infectious, inflammatory rashes).
2. Therapeutic removal of symptomatic benign lesions when appropriate.
3. Note: If melanoma is suspected, prefer an excisional biopsy with narrow margins when feasible.

CONTRAINDICATIONS

1. Overlying cellulitis/active infection at site (choose alternative site or delay if possible).
2. True allergy to local anesthetic.
3. Uncorrected coagulopathy/anticoagulation with high bleeding risk (weigh risks/benefits; apply meticulous hemostasis).
4. Relative: suspected melanoma (avoid superficial shave), cosmetically sensitive areas,

poor wound healing risk (e.g., severe PVD on distal sites).

CONSENT

1. Purpose: obtain tissue for histopathology ± remove lesion; may require additional treatment based on results.
2. Benefits: diagnostic clarity and potential symptom relief.
3. Risks: bleeding/hematoma, infection, pain, scarring/keloid, pigment change, nerve injury (rare), incomplete sampling requiring re-biopsy.
4. Alternatives: clinical/dermoscopic monitoring, imaging if indicated, referral for excisional biopsy.

PREPARATION

1. Confirm lesion/site and take photo/diagram; mark margins/orientation if needed.
2. Asepsis: cleanse with chlorhexidine or povidone-iodine; sterile gloves for punch/excision.
3. Local anesthesia: 1% lidocaine ± epinephrine (avoid epinephrine based on local protocol for end-artery areas).
4. Check meds (anticoagulants) and allergies; gather equipment and labeled formalin container.

EQUIPMENT

1. Antiseptic swabs, sterile gloves, gauze, adhesive

bandage.

2. Syringe with 25–30G needle; 1% lidocaine ± epinephrine.

3. Shave blade/dermaplane or #15 blade; punch tools (2–6 mm).

4. Adson forceps (toothed), iris scissors.

5. Hemostasis: direct pressure, aluminum chloride (20–40%), silver nitrate (avoid near eyes).

6. Suture material (4-0 to 6-0 nylon) for punch ≥3–4 mm or under tension.

7. Pre-labeled formalin jar; pathology requisition (include site, differential, orientation).

PROCEDURE STEPS — SHAVE BIOPSY (TANGENTIAL)

1. Indications: raised benign-appearing lesions (e.g., seborrheic keratosis), superficial NMSC suspicion; not for suspected melanoma.

2. Anesthetize. Hold blade parallel to skin; shave through epidermis/superficial dermis to remove lesion with a thin disc.

3. Achieve hemostasis (aluminum chloride/ pressure). Place specimen in formalin; label with site.

4. Apply petrolatum and dressing.

PROCEDURE STEPS — PUNCH BIOPSY (FULL-THICKNESS CORE)

1. Indications: inflammatory rashes, small lesions, or when depth is needed. For pigmented lesions where excision not feasible, perform deep punch to subcutis.

2. Select size: 3–4 mm for rashes; 4–6 mm for neoplasms. Stretch skin perpendicular to relaxed skin tension lines to create an ellipse.

3. Advance punch with gentle rotation to subcutis. Lift core minimally with forceps; snip base with scissors.

4. Close with simple interrupted sutures if needed; otherwise allow to heal by secondary intention depending on size/site.

SPECIMEN HANDLING

1. Place in formalin immediately (do NOT use formalin if sending for culture/direct immunofluorescence—use appropriate media).

2. Label with patient, exact site, and orientation (mark tip/suture if needed).

3. Complete requisition: site, clinical description, duration, differential, prior treatments, and special tests requested.

COMPLICATIONS / SIDE EFFECTS

1. Bleeding/hematoma, infection, pain.
2. Scar, hypertrophic/keloid scar risk (sternum, shoulders, upper back, deltoid).
3. Dyspigmentation, wound dehiscence.
4. Rare: nerve injury, allergic reaction to anesthetic, granulation tissue.

AFTERCARE & MONITORING

1. Keep dressing dry 24 h; then daily gentle cleanse, petrolatum, and fresh dressing until epithelialized.
2. Analgesia: acetaminophen/NSAIDs if appropriate.
3. Red flags: increasing pain, erythema, warmth, purulent discharge, fever, numbness.
4. Suture removal (typical): face 5–7 d; scalp 7–10 d; trunk/upper limb 10–14 d; lower limb 12–14 d.
5. Arrange result follow-up and plan for definitive management if malignancy is found.

DISPOSITION

1. Discharge with wound care instructions and clear follow-up for pathology results (usually 7–14 days).
2. Escalate/urgent referral if melanoma/invasive carcinoma suspected or margins positive requiring wider excision.

REFERENCES

NHS — Skin biopsy (patient guidance). https://www. nhs.uk

DermNet NZ — Skin biopsy: indications and techniques. https://dermnetnz.org

MyHealth.Alberta.ca — Skin biopsy: what to expect at home. https://myhealth.alberta.ca

Cancer Research UK — Skin biopsies for melanoma and skin cancer (patient info). https:// www.cancerresearchuk.org

HealthLink BC — Minor skin procedures and wound care (patient info). https://www.healthlinkbc.ca

EXCISIONAL BIOPSY
(ELLIPTICAL) — SKIN LESIONS

INDICATIONS

1. Suspicious pigmented or non-pigmented skin lesions where complete sampling is preferred (e.g., melanoma suspicion, atypical nevi, NMSC).
2. Small lesions where full removal with narrow margins is feasible for diagnosis and treatment.
3. Recurrent or changing lesions where prior partial biopsy was non-diagnostic.

CONTRAINDICATIONS

1. Overlying cellulitis/active infection at site (delay if possible or choose alternate site).
2. Uncorrected coagulopathy with high bleeding risk; consider optimization and meticulous hemostasis.
3. Relative: cosmetically critical sites (e.g., central face) — consider referral; lesions requiring complex reconstruction.

CONSENT

4. Purpose: complete removal of lesion for histopathology with orientation of margins.
5. Benefits: definitive diagnosis, often therapeutic for benign/NMSC lesions; accurate Breslow depth in melanoma.
6. Risks: bleeding/hematoma, infection, scarring/ keloid or dyspigmentation, wound dehiscence, nerve injury (site-dependent), need for wider excision if malignancy confirmed.

PREPARATION

1. Confirm lesion/site with patient; mark along relaxed skin tension lines; photograph/diagram if helpful.
2. Skin antisepsis (chlorhexidine or povidone-iodine); sterile field and gloves.
3. Local anesthesia: 1% lidocaine ± epinephrine (avoid epinephrine in end-artery areas per local protocol).
4. Plan ellipse length-to-width ~3:1; apices ~30° to reduce dog-ears. Consider marking orientation (e.g., superior = single suture, lateral = double).

EQUIPMENT

1. Antiseptic swabs, sterile gloves, drapes, gauze.
2. Syringe with 25–30G needle; local anesthetic.
3. Scalpel (#15), Adson forceps (toothed), iris/

metzenbaum scissors.

4. Needle driver, hemostats; electrocautery or aluminum chloride/silver nitrate for hemostasis as appropriate.

5. Suture material: deep dermal absorbable 4-0/5-0; epidermal nylon/prolene 4-0/5-0 (face 5-0/6-0).

6. Specimen container with formalin (or appropriate medium if special studies are planned). Pathology requisition.

MARGINS & ORIENTATION (DIAGNOSIS-FOCUSED)

1. For suspected melanoma: excise with **narrow clinical margins (1–3 mm)** down to subcutaneous fat to permit accurate Breslow depth (definitive wider excision follows pathology).

2. For NMSC or benign lesions where diagnostic excision is intended, use conservative margins per local guidance.

3. Mark orientation with sutures/ink (e.g., long stitch superior, short stitch lateral). Communicate suspected diagnosis and lesion map on requisition.

PROCEDURE STEPS — ELLIPTICAL EXCISION

1. Infiltrate anesthetic around (not through) the lesion; allow time for effect.
2. Incise the outlined ellipse perpendicular to skin; include full thickness to subcutis.
3. Undermine minimally (2–5 mm) in the superficial subcutis to reduce tension while preserving vessels.
4. Achieve hemostasis (pressure/electrocautery/ chemical).
5. Close in layers: deep dermal interrupted sutures to relieve tension; then simple interrupted or running epidermal sutures along tension lines.
6. Place orientation sutures on the specimen, confirm labels, and transfer to formalin promptly.

SPECIMEN HANDLING

1. Label container with patient details, exact site, and orientation key; include clinical description, differential, and prior biopsies.
2. Do **not** place in formalin if direct immunofluorescence or culture is required—use appropriate media and separate requisitions.

COMPLICATIONS / SIDE EFFECTS

1. Bleeding/hematoma, infection, pain.
2. Scar, hypertrophic/keloid risk (shoulders, chest, upper back).
3. Dyspigmentation, wound dehiscence; rare nerve injury depending on site.

AFTERCARE & MONITORING

1. Keep dressing dry 24 h; then gentle daily cleansing, petrolatum, and new dressing until epithelialized.
2. Activity: avoid tension on the wound; consider steri-strips after suture removal if under tension.
3. Suture removal (typical): face 5–7 d; scalp 7–10 d; trunk/upper limb 10–14 d; lower limb 12–14 d.
4. Red flags: increasing pain, erythema, warmth, purulent drainage, fever, numbness/weakness.

DISPOSITION

1. Discharge with wound care and ensure pathology follow-up (7–14 days).
2. If melanoma/NMSC confirmed, arrange guideline-directed wider excision and staging/ referral as indicated.

REFERENCES

NHS — Skin biopsy and excision: patient guidance. https://www.nhs.uk

DermNet NZ — Excision of skin lesions and surgical techniques. https://dermnetnz.org

Cancer Research UK — Skin cancer biopsies and excisions (patient info). https://www.cancerresearchuk.org

MyHealth.Alberta.ca — Skin excision: care instructions. https://myhealth.alberta.ca

HealthLink BC — Minor skin procedures and wound care (patient info). https://www.healthlinkbc.ca

EPIDERMOID ("SEBACEOUS") CYST

—

INCISION & DRAINAGE ± EXCISION

INDICATIONS

1. Symptomatic cyst causing pain, recurrent swelling/infection, rupture/drainage, or functional/cosmetic concern.

2. Fluctuant, infected cyst requiring abscess drainage.

3. Diagnostic uncertainty or atypical features (consider histopathology).

CONTRAINDICATIONS

1. Overlying cellulitis without abscess—optimize antibiotics first unless urgent drainage needed.

2. True allergy to local anesthetic.

3. Relative: anticoagulation/coagulopathy (use meticulous hemostasis), acutely inflamed cyst for elective excision (defer until quiescent), lesions in cosmetically sensitive/nerve-dense areas (consider referral).

CONSENT

1. Purpose: drain infection and/or remove cyst; recurrence risk discussed (higher if capsule not completely removed).

2. Benefits: pain relief, infection control, definitive removal when excised.

3. Risks: bleeding/hematoma, infection, scarring/ dyspigmentation, wound dehiscence, nerve injury (site dependent), recurrence (especially after I&D alone).

4. Alternatives: observation (if asymptomatic), antibiotics when indicated, referral for surgical removal.

PREPARATION

1. Confirm site and mark along relaxed skin tension lines; identify punctum if present.

2. Asepsis: chlorhexidine or povidone–iodine; sterile gloves and small drape.

3. Local anesthesia: 1% lidocaine ± epinephrine per local protocol; avoid epi in end-artery areas as per local guidance.

4. Consider ultrasound if diagnosis uncertain or near critical structures.

EQUIPMENT

1. Antiseptic swabs, sterile gloves, gauze, adhesive dressing.

2. Syringe with 25–30G needle; local anesthetic.
3. Scalpel (#11 for I&D; #15 for excision), hemostats, blunt scissors, curette.
4. Irrigation (saline), hemostasis agents (pressure, aluminum chloride; cautery if available).
5. Suture material (4-0/5-0 nylon) for excision closure; specimen container with formalin if sending tissue.

PROCEDURE — INCISION & DRAINAGE (INFECTED/FLUCTUANT CYST)

1. Incise over point of maximal fluctuance along skin lines; express keratinous material and pus.
2. Break loculations with hemostat/curette; irrigate thoroughly.
3. Consider loose packing or wick for 24–48 h if cavity large; otherwise leave open to drain.
4. Antibiotics only if surrounding cellulitis, systemic symptoms, or high-risk patient per local guidance.

PROCEDURE — ELECTIVE EXCISION (QUIESCENT/NON-INFLAMED CYST)

1. Outline an ellipse including the punctum; infiltrate field with local anesthetic.
2. Incise through dermis to cyst wall; perform gentle blunt dissection around capsule, avoiding rupture.

3. Deliver cyst intact if possible; if rupture occurs, remove all capsule remnants to reduce recurrence.

4. Achieve hemostasis; close in layers (deep dermal as needed, then skin). Send specimen if atypical.

COMPLICATIONS / SIDE EFFECTS

1. Recurrence (especially after I&D only or incomplete capsule removal).

2. Infection, bleeding/hematoma, scarring/keloid, dyspigmentation.

3. Wound dehiscence, nerve injury (site dependent).

AFTERCARE & MONITORING

1. I&D: daily dressing changes; remove packing in 24–48 h; warm compresses; return if fever, spreading erythema, increasing pain.

2. Excision: keep dressing dry 24 h; then cleanse daily, petrolatum, new dressing. Suture removal: face 5–7 d; scalp 7–10 d; trunk/upper limb 10–14 d; lower limb 12–14 d.

3. Arrange follow-up for wound review and pathology (if sent).

DISPOSITION

1. Discharge with written wound care and red-flag instructions; arrange follow-up.
2. Refer for surgical/dermatology evaluation if recurrent, large, atypical, or in high-risk locations.

REFERENCES

NHS — Epidermoid (sebaceous) cyst: overview and treatment. https://www.nhs.uk

DermNet NZ — Epidermoid cyst (sebaceous cyst): diagnosis and management. https://dermnetnz.org

MyHealth.Alberta.ca — Skin abscess and cyst care instructions. https://myhealth.alberta.ca

HealthLink BC — Minor skin procedures and wound care (patient info). https://www.healthlinkbc.ca

American Academy of Dermatology (AAD) — Epidermoid cysts (patient information). https://www.aad.org

LIPOMA — OFFICE EXCISION

INDICATIONS

1. Symptomatic subcutaneous mass (pain, irritation, recurrent trauma) or cosmetic concern.
2. Documented growth or functional limitation.
3. Diagnostic uncertainty after clinical/ultrasound exam — excision for histopathology.

RED FLAGS (CONSIDER IMAGING/ REFERRAL, NOT OFFICE EXCISION)

1. >5 cm, rapidly enlarging, firm/fixed or deep to fascia.
2. Overlying skin changes, neurovascular proximity, or atypical features suggesting liposarcoma.
3. Recurrence after prior excision.

CONTRAINDICATIONS

1. Overlying cellulitis/active infection.
2. Uncorrected coagulopathy or high bleeding risk (relative).
3. Lesions in high-risk/cosmetically critical areas

(face, hands, near major nerves/vessels) — consider referral.

CONSENT

1. Purpose: remove lesion and obtain diagnosis.
2. Benefits: symptom relief, definitive treatment, pathology confirmation.
3. Risks: bleeding/hematoma, infection, scarring/contour defect, seroma, nerve injury (site-dependent), recurrence.
4. Alternatives: observation, imaging, specialist referral.

PREPARATION

1. Confirm site with patient; mark along relaxed skin tension lines.
2. Asepsis: chlorhexidine or povidone-iodine; sterile drape and gloves.
3. Local anesthetic: 1% lidocaine ± epinephrine per local protocol (avoid epi in end-artery areas per local guidance).
4. Consider ultrasound if depth/planes uncertain.

EQUIPMENT

1. Antiseptic swabs, sterile gloves, drapes, gauze.
2. Syringe with 25–27G needle; local anesthetic.
3. Scalpel (#15), Adson forceps (toothed), Metzenbaum scissors, hemostats.

4. Blunt dissection tool (peanut/gauze; curved mosquito).

5. Hemostasis: pressure, aluminum chloride, cautery if available.

6. Suture: deep dermal absorbable (4-0/5-0) and skin nylon/prolene (4-0/5-0).

7. Specimen container with formalin; pathology requisition.

PROCEDURE — ELLIPTICAL EXCISION WITH BLUNT DISSECTION

1. Infiltrate anesthetic around lesion; allow time for effect.

2. Make a skin incision over the lipoma along tension lines, sized to permit delivery without undue force.

3. Carry dissection through dermis to the lipoma capsule. Use blunt dissection and traction–counter-traction to free the encapsulated mass circumferentially.

4. Control perforating vessels with pressure/cautery. Avoid injury to nearby sensory nerves.

5. Deliver the lipoma intact. Inspect cavity; excise residual lobules if present.

6. Irrigate, achieve hemostasis, and consider small closed-space dead-space reduction with a few deep dermal sutures.

7. Close skin with simple interrupted or running

sutures; consider subcuticular closure for cosmesis.

SPECIMEN HANDLING

1. Place entire lesion in formalin. Label with patient data, exact site, and clinical notes (size, duration, growth).
2. Request histopathology for confirmation; note any atypical features.

COMPLICATIONS / SIDE EFFECTS

1. Bleeding/hematoma, infection, seroma, contour defect.
2. Scar, hypertrophic/keloid risk (shoulders, chest, back).
3. Nerve irritation/numbness (site-dependent), recurrence if residual tissue remains.

AFTERCARE & MONITORING

1. Keep dressing dry 24 h; then daily gentle cleanse, petrolatum, and fresh dressing.
2. Activity: avoid tension/pressure on the site for several days.
3. Suture removal (typical): trunk/upper limb 10–14 d; lower limb 12–14 d; scalp 7–10 d; face 5–7 d.
4. Return precautions: increasing pain, redness, warmth, purulent drainage, fever, expanding hematoma.

DISPOSITION

1. Discharge with wound care instructions and follow-up for pathology results (7–14 d).
2. Refer if histology unexpected or margins unclear, or if recurrence occurs.

REFERENCES

NHS — Lipoma: overview and treatment. https://www.nhs.uk

DermNet NZ — Lipoma: clinical features and management. https://dermnetnz.org

American Academy of Dermatology (AAD) — Lipoma (patient information). https://www.aad.org

MyHealth.Alberta.ca — Skin excision/aftercare. https://myhealth.alberta.ca

HealthLink BC — Minor skin procedures and wound care (patient info). https://www.healthlinkbc.ca

CRYOTHERAPY — COMMON & PLANTAR WARTS (VERRUCA)

INDICATIONS

1. Symptomatic or persistent common/plantar warts (pain, functional/cosmetic impact).
2. Periungual/filiform warts where precise application feasible.
3. Consider in pregnancy if treatment required (no teratogenic risk from LN2).

CONTRAINDICATIONS / CAUTIONS

1. Suspected skin cancer or uncertain diagnosis — do **not** freeze; biopsy/refer.
2. Cold intolerance disorders: cryoglobulinemia, cold urticaria, Raynaud phenomenon; severe peripheral vascular disease/neuropathy (digits).
3. Darkly pigmented skin (higher dyspigmentation risk), poor wound healing, anticoagulation (bleeding/blister size).
4. Caution near nail matrix, over tendons/nerve-rich areas, or in patients with lymphedema.

CONSENT

1. Purpose: destroy wart tissue via freeze–thaw injury.

2. Benefits: clearance or debulking; can combine with keratolytics and debridement.

3. Risks: pain, blister/edema, infection, **hypo/hyperpigmentation**, scarring, nail dystrophy (periungual), nerve injury (rare).

4. Alternatives: watchful waiting, salicylic acid, cantharidin (if available), curettage, immunotherapy, laser.

PREPARATION

1. Confirm diagnosis. Pare thick hyperkeratosis (plantar) with curette/scalpel to improve freeze depth.

2. Clean with alcohol/chlorhexidine; consider topical/local anesthesia for sensitive sites/children.

3. Protect surrounding skin with petrolatum if needed.

EQUIPMENT

1. Liquid nitrogen (LN_2) cryospray gun **or** cotton-tip/dipstick applicator; appropriate cones/shields.

2. Gauze, forceps/curette, petrolatum, dressings; optional eye protection for operator/patient.

TECHNIQUE — TYPICAL FREEZE TIMES

1. Aim for **1–2 mm ice halo** beyond lesion (up to 2–3 mm for plantar).
2. Common warts: **10–20 s freeze**, **1–2 cycles**; allow full thaw between cycles.
3. Plantar warts: **20–40 s freeze**, **2 cycles** after paring callus.
4. Filiform/periungual: shorter controlled bursts; avoid nail matrix; consider multiple short sprays.
5. Repeat sessions every **2–3 weeks** until resolution (typically 2–4 visits).

COMPLICATIONS / SIDE EFFECTS

1. Pain during/after, blister/serous or hemorrhagic bulla, edema, temporary loss of function (foot).
2. Dyspigmentation (more in darker skin), scarring/atrophy, nail dystrophy, neuropathic pain (rare).
3. Infection (impetigo/cellulitis) — uncommon.

AFTERCARE & MONITORING

1. Expect blister/erythema in 6–24 h; keep clean/dry 24 h then daily gentle wash; petrolatum and dressing as needed.
2. Elevation/analgesics PRN; offload plantar lesions. Do not intentionally deroof blisters unless tense/painful (sterile drainage).
3. Adjunct: daily **salicylic acid** between sessions for plantar warts if skin tolerates.

4. Return if spreading erythema, fever, pus, or severe pain; reassess after 2–3 weeks.

DISPOSITION

1. Stop after 3–4 unsuccessful treatments; consider alternative modalities or referral.

REFERENCES

DermNet NZ — Warts (Verrucae) & Cryotherapy: indications/technique. https://dermnetnz.org

NHS — Warts and verrucas: treatment. https://www.nhs.uk

American Academy of Dermatology — Warts: diagnosis and treatment (patient info). https://www.aad.org

American Family Physician — Treatment of Nongenital Cutaneous Warts (open access). https://www.aafp.org

MyHealth.Alberta.ca — Warts care instructions. https://myhealth.alberta.ca

CRYOTHERAPY — ACTINIC KERATOSIS (AK)

INDICATIONS

1. Clinically diagnosed isolated AKs, especially hyperkeratotic lesions not suited to field therapy.
2. Symptomatic (tender) or cosmetically concerning AKs.
3. Patients preferring procedural treatment vs. topical field therapies.

CONTRAINDICATIONS / CAUTIONS

1. Uncertain diagnosis or features suspicious for SCC in situ/invasive SCC — biopsy first.
2. Extensive field disease better managed with field therapy (5-FU, imiquimod, PDT) — consider combination approach.
3. Cold-sensitivity disorders (cryoglobulinemia, cold urticaria, Raynaud), poor wound healing, darker skin (dyspigmentation risk).

CONSENT

1. Purpose: targeted destruction of AK by freeze–thaw injury.

2. Benefits: high clearance for thin lesions, quick in-office.

3. Risks: pain, blister/crust, **hypo/hyperpigmentation**, atrophy/scar (especially with long freezes), infection.

4. Alternatives: emollients/observation, curettage, field therapies (5-FU/imiquimod), photodynamic therapy, excision if diagnostic doubt.

PREPARATION

1. Confirm AK clinically/dermoscopically; pare hyperkeratosis to improve freeze penetration.

2. Clean skin; protect surrounding skin with petrolatum if needed.

EQUIPMENT

1. LN$_2$ cryospray gun or cotton-tip/dipstick; cones/shields; gauze and dressings.

TECHNIQUE — TYPICAL FREEZE TIMES

1. Thin AK: **5–10 s single freeze** aiming for **1–2 mm halo**.

2. Thick/hyperkeratotic AK: **10–20 s**, may use **1–2 cycles** after paring.

3. Lips (actinic cheilitis) generally not treated with standard spray in primary care — refer for field therapy/PDT unless experienced.

COMPLICATIONS / SIDE EFFECTS

1. Pain, edema/erythema, blister/crust forming in 24–48 h.
2. Dyspigmentation (common in darker skin), atrophy/scar with aggressive freezing.
3. Infection is uncommon.

AFTERCARE & MONITORING

1. Clean daily after 24 h; petrolatum + dressing until crust separates (1–3 weeks depending on site).
2. Sun protection; treat additional field disease as appropriate.
3. Reassess non-healing lesions (>8 weeks) or recurrent/thickening lesions for biopsy.

REFERENCES

DermNet NZ — Actinic keratosis and cryotherapy. https://dermnetnz.org

Cancer Research UK — Actinic keratosis treatment options. https://www.cancerresearchuk.org

NHS — Actinic keratoses (solar keratoses): treatment. https://www.nhs.uk

American Family Physician — Cutaneous Cryosurgery for Common Skin Conditions (open access). https://www.aafp.org

MyHealth.Alberta.ca — Actinic keratosis care. https://myhealth.alberta.ca

CRYOTHERAPY — OTHER BENIGN LESIONS (SEBORRHEIC KERATOSIS, SKIN TAGS, MOLLUSCUM)

INDICATIONS

1. Clinically benign lesions diagnosed with confidence: seborrheic keratoses (SK), acrochordons (skin tags), molluscum contagiosum.
2. Symptomatic (irritation/trauma) or cosmetic concerns after discussing risks.

CONTRAINDICATIONS / CAUTIONS

1. Atypical pigmented or changing lesions — **do not** freeze; consider biopsy.
2. Facial cosmetically sensitive areas and darker skin types (higher dyspigmentation risk) — consider alternative methods/test spot.
3. Periocular/perioral areas, genital lesions (specialist). Cold sensitivity disorders as above.

CONSENT

1. Purpose: lesion destruction for symptom/ cosmesis.

2. Benefits: quick office treatment; often hemostatic.

3. Risks: pain, blister/crust, **hypo/ hyperpigmentation** (common), atrophy/scar, milia, alopecia in hair-bearing skin.

4. Alternatives: curettage/shave for SK, snip excision for tags, watchful waiting for molluscum (self-limited).

PREPARATION

1. Confirm benign diagnosis; document size/site; photograph if cosmetic.

2. Clean skin; consider petrolatum barrier around lesion.

EQUIPMENT

1. LN$_2$ cryospray or cotton-tip/dipstick; cones/ shields; gauze and dressings.

TECHNIQUE — TYPICAL FREEZE TIMES

1. Seborrheic keratosis: **5–10 s** (thin) to **10–15 s** (thick), **1–2 cycles**; or consider curettage.

2. Skin tags: brief touch freeze **1–3 s**, usually single cycle; alternative is snip/excision with hemostasis.

3. Molluscum: **1–5 s** light freeze to avoid scarring; consider limited test area; repeat every

2–3 weeks as needed.

COMPLICATIONS / SIDE EFFECTS

1. Pain, blister, crust; dyspigmentation (common), atrophy/scar, milia, alopecia.
2. Secondary infection is uncommon.

AFTERCARE & MONITORING

1. Daily gentle cleansing after 24 h; petrolatum until healed. Avoid picking/sun exposure; use sunscreen.
2. Reassess if lesion persists >8 weeks or changes atypically — consider biopsy/shave/curettage.

REFERENCES

DermNet NZ — Seborrhoeic keratosis; Molluscum; Skin tag; Cryotherapy. https://dermnetnz.org

NHS — Seborrhoeic keratoses and skin tags: treatment. https://www.nhs.uk

American Academy of Dermatology — Molluscum & SK patient info. https://www.aad.org

American Family Physician — Cutaneous Cryosurgery for Common Skin Conditions (open access). https://www.aafp.org

MyHealth.Alberta.ca — Skin lesion care after treatment. https://myhealth.alberta.ca

GENITAL WARTS (ANOGENITAL HPV) — RYOTHERAPY & MEDICAL TREATMENTS

INDICATIONS

1. Symptomatic anogenital warts (pain, itch, bleeding, psychosocial distress) on external genitalia/perineum/perianal skin.
2. Patient preference for removal or reduction of visible warts.
3. Note: Treatment is **not required** for asymptomatic lesions; spontaneous regression occurs in some cases.

CONTRAINDICATIONS / CAUTIONS

1. Uncertain diagnosis or suspicious lesion (ulcerated, pigmented, rapidly growing) — **biopsy/refer** before treatment.
2. Pregnancy: **avoid podophyllotoxin/podophyllin and sinecatechins**. Cryotherapy or TCA/BCA are acceptable options.
3. Urethral meatus, vaginal/cervical canal, or

anal canal involvement — consider specialist management.

4. Immunocompromised (incl. HIV): higher recurrence; consider earlier specialist referral.

CONSENT

1. Purpose: remove or reduce visible warts and associated symptoms; does **not** eradicate HPV.

2. Benefits: symptom relief, improved cosmesis, fewer visible lesions.

3. Risks: pain, blister/ulceration, infection, **dyspigmentation** or scarring, sexual discomfort, recurrence (common).

4. Alternatives: observation, different treatment modality, or referral.

PREPARATION

1. Confirm pregnancy status where relevant; offer **STI screening** including HIV and syphilis per local guidance.

2. Discuss HPV vaccination (catch-up as eligible).

3. For cryotherapy: pare hyperkeratotic lesions; protect surrounding skin with petrolatum if needed.

FIRST-LINE TREATMENT OPTIONS (EXTERNAL GENITAL/PERIANAL SKIN)

1. **Cryotherapy (LN_2, clinician-applied):** Spray or probe until **ice halo 1–2 mm** beyond lesion. Typical **10–20 s freeze**, allow full thaw; **1–2 cycles** per session. Repeat every **1–2 weeks** until clearance.

2. **Trichloroacetic or Bichloroacetic Acid 80–90% (clinician-applied):** Small amount to each wart until frosting; **once weekly**; neutralize with sodium bicarbonate or soap/water if excess spread.

3. **Imiquimod 5% cream (patient-applied):** Thin layer **3 nights/week** (e.g., Mon/Wed/Fri) at bedtime, wash off after **6–10 h**; continue up to **16 weeks**. (3.75% formulation: **nightly** up to **8 weeks**.)

4. **Podofilox/Podophyllotoxin 0.5% (patient-applied):** Apply **BID for 3 days**, then **4 days off**; repeat up to **4 cycles**. Limit area (**≤10 cm²**) and volume (**≤0.5 mL/day**). **Avoid in pregnancy.**

5. **Sinecatechins 15% ointment (patient-applied):** Apply **TID** until clearance for up to **16 weeks**; do **not** wash off after application. **Avoid in pregnancy and immunocompromise.**

SPECIAL SITES / WHEN TO REFER

1. Meatal, urethral, vaginal, cervical, or intra-anal warts; large or obstructive lesions; failure of multiple modalities; severe immunosuppression.

2. Surgical options (specialist): curettage/shave, electrosurgery, CO_2 laser, excision — useful for bulky or refractory lesions.

CRYOTHERAPY — QUICK TECHNIQUE

1. Dry skin; shield mucosa. Apply LN_2 until a thin **1–2 mm halo** forms. For thicker lesions, consider **two freeze–thaw cycles** (10–20 s each).

2. Expect blister/erosion; avoid overlapping fields to reduce scarring; space sessions **1–2 weeks**.

3. Pain control: topical anesthetic, oral analgesics; warn about transient swelling and exudate.

TOPICALS — KEY SAFETY POINTS

1. Avoid sexual contact while medication is on the skin; **condoms reduce but don't eliminate** HPV transmission.

2. Wash hands after application; avoid occlusion unless directed.

3. Stop and seek review for severe irritation, ulceration, or systemic symptoms.

AFTERCARE & MONITORING

1. Clean gently daily; petrolatum and non-adherent dressing for erosions. Expect crusting/blister for 1–7 days post-cryo.

2. Advise no picking/shaving over treated area; abstain or use barrier protection until healed and medication washed off.

3. Reassess in **2–3 months**; recurrence is common, especially in first year. Consider switching modality if inadequate response.

PATIENT EDUCATION

1. HPV often persists subclinically; visible wart removal does **not** guarantee non-infectivity.

2. Offer/advise HPV vaccination per age/eligibility; discuss partner notification/testing as appropriate.

3. Screen for cervical cancer per guidelines; manage anxiety and stigma empathetically.

REFERENCES

Centers for Disease Control and Prevention (CDC) — 2021 STI Treatment Guidelines: Anogenital Warts. https://www.cdc.gov

World Health Organization (WHO) — HPV and anogenital warts management resources (open access). https://www.who.int

British Association for Sexual Health and HIV (BASHH) — 2015/updated guidance on management of anogenital warts (open access). https://www.bashh.org

NHS — Genital warts: treatment options. https://www.nhs.uk

Healthdirect Australia — Genital warts. https://www.healthdirect.gov.au

MyHealth.Alberta.ca — Genital warts: care instructions. https://myhealth.alberta.ca

NAIL/HAND INFECTIONS & NAILBED CARE

INGROWN TOENAIL — PARTIAL NAIL AVULSION (± CHEMICAL MATRIXECTOMY)

INDICATIONS

1. Painful onychocryptosis (Grade II–III) with granulation/secondary infection or recurrent episodes.
2. Failure of conservative care (soaks, cotton/gutter splint, footwear changes).
3. Significant functional impairment or deforming nail edge.

CONTRAINDICATIONS

1. Absolute: suspected osteomyelitis, spreading cellulitis with systemic illness (manage first).
2. Relative: severe peripheral arterial disease/poor wound healing, uncontrolled diabetes, coagulopathy/anticoagulation, allergy to anesthetic or phenol, pregnancy (avoid phenol per local protocol).

CONSENT

1. Purpose: remove offending nail edge; optional chemical ablation of ipsilateral matrix to reduce recurrence.
2. Benefits: pain relief, faster resolution, lower recurrence with matrixectomy.
3. Risks: bleeding, infection, delayed healing (longer with phenol), recurrence/spicule formation, nail dystrophy, chemical burn to surrounding skin, transient numbness/paresthesia.

PREPARATION

1. Confirm digit and side; assess vascular status and infection severity; mark site.
2. Asepsis: chlorhexidine or povidone-iodine; sterile gloves and small drape.
3. Digital block: 1% lidocaine ± epinephrine as permitted by local protocol (avoid epinephrine in end-artery digits if required).
4. Apply digital tourniquet (penrose/elastic) at base of toe; prep dry field.

EQUIPMENT

1. Antiseptic swabs, sterile gloves, gauze, small sterile drape, adhesive dressing.
2. Syringe (5–10 mL) with 25–27G needle; local anesthetic.
3. Nail elevator/freer, straight hemostat, nail splitter

or iris scissors.

4. Curette for granulation tissue; silver nitrate stick (optional).

5. Phenol 80–88% with cotton-tipped applicators (if performing matrixectomy); copious saline for irrigation.

6. Petrolatum and non-adherent dressing; toe spacer/cotton if desired.

PROCEDURE — PARTIAL NAIL AVULSION (LATERAL EDGE)

1. Lift lateral nail edge with elevator; free from lateral nail fold to the matrix.

2. Create a longitudinal cut 3–4 mm from nail edge through to the matrix with nail splitter/scissors.

3. Grasp the strip with hemostat and remove in one piece by rolling outward; ensure removal back to the matrix horn.

4. Debride exuberant granulation tissue; achieve hemostasis (pressure ± silver nitrate).

OPTIONAL — CHEMICAL MATRIXECTOMY (TO REDUCE RECURRENCE)

1. Dry the field. Protect surrounding skin with petrolatum.

2. Apply 80–88% phenol on cotton-tipped applicator to exposed lateral matrix for 30 seconds × 2–3

applications using fresh swabs each time.

3. Irrigate thoroughly with saline to dilute/clear phenol; remove tourniquet.

COMPLICATIONS / SIDE EFFECTS

1. Infection, delayed healing (more common with phenol), bleeding/hematoma.

2. Recurrence or spicule formation if matrix not fully ablated.

3. Chemical burn/skin necrosis from phenol contact; nail dystrophy, pain flare.

4. Rare: allergic reaction, persistent numbness.

AFTERCARE & MONITORING

1. Keep dressing dry 24–48 h; then daily warm saline soaks, dry, petrolatum, and fresh non-adherent dressing until healed.

2. Relative rest/elevation 24–48 h; roomy footwear or open-toe sandal.

3. Analgesia: acetaminophen/NSAIDs if appropriate.

4. Red flags: increasing pain, spreading erythema, purulent drainage, fever, or progressive numbness.

5. Antibiotics only if cellulitis/systemic signs per local guidance; schedule review in 1–2 weeks.

DISPOSITION

1. Discharge with written aftercare; advise recurrence risk and when to return.
2. Consider podiatry/dermatology/orthopedics referral for atypical cases or recurrent failures.

REFERENCES

NHS — Ingrown toenail: treatment. https://www.nhs.uk

NICE CKS — Ingrowing toenails (open access). https://cks.nice.org.uk

HealthLink BC — Ingrown toenail care. https://www.healthlinkbc.ca

MyHealth.Alberta.ca — Ingrown toenail: care instructions. https://myhealth.alberta.ca

Healthdirect Australia — Ingrown toenail: treatment and self-care. https://www.healthdirect.gov.au

American Orthopaedic Foot & Ankle Society (AOFAS) — Ingrown toenails (patient education). https://www.aofas.org

PARONYCHIA — INCISION & DRAINAGE (I&D)

INDICATIONS

1. Acute painful swelling and fluctuance at the nail fold (finger or toe).
2. Failure of conservative care (soaks, elevation, antibiotics when indicated).
3. Diagnostic relief of abscess; obtain sample if unusual organisms suspected.

CONTRAINDICATIONS / SPECIAL CONSIDERATIONS

1. Suspected **herpetic whitlow** (vesicles, severe pain) — **do not incise**; manage conservatively.
2. Felon (pulp space abscess) requires different incision approach — consider referral.
3. Overlying cellulitis without abscess — treat medically first unless evolving abscess.
4. Relative: severe peripheral arterial disease, coagulopathy/anticoagulation, allergy to anesthetic.

CONSENT

1. Purpose: drain abscess to relieve pain and promote healing.
2. Benefits: rapid symptom relief and shorter illness duration.
3. Risks: bleeding, infection spread, nail dystrophy, soft-tissue injury, recurrence, scarring, rare nerve injury.
4. Alternatives: continued conservative care (soaks), antibiotics if cellulitis/systemic signs, delayed I&D if early.

PREPARATION

1. Confirm digit and side; assess for felon or whitlow; check tetanus status if trauma.
2. Asepsis: chlorhexidine or povidone-iodine; sterile gloves and small drape.
3. Digital block with 1% lidocaine (no epinephrine if your local protocol advises against it); allow time for anesthesia.
4. Apply a digital tourniquet (penrose/elastic) for a dry field.

EQUIPMENT

1. Antiseptic swabs, sterile gloves, gauze, small sterile drape, adhesive dressing.
2. Syringe (5–10 mL) with 25–27G needle; 1% lidocaine.

3. No. 11 blade; small blunt elevator/freer or hypodermic needle for lifting nail fold.

4. Irrigation (saline); cotton/ribbon gauze or small wick; forceps, hemostat.

5. Optional: culture swab if atypical/infected bite or water exposure; antibiotics per local guidance if cellulitis/systemic signs.

PROCEDURE STEPS — SIMPLE PARONYCHIA (LATERAL NAIL FOLD)

1. Prep and drape. Identify area of maximal fluctuance at the lateral nail fold.

2. Using the tip of a No. 11 blade or a blunt-tipped instrument, gently elevate the lateral nail fold off the nail plate to allow pus to egress **(preferred minimal-incision technique)**.

3. If required, make a **small longitudinal stab incision** parallel to the nail edge at the nail fold (avoid crossing into nail bed).

4. Express and irrigate the cavity thoroughly with saline until clear.

5. If the abscess tracks beneath the nail edge, **lift or remove a thin lateral strip of nail** (2–3 mm) to permit drainage back to the matrix horn.

6. Place a small wick (plain gauze) to keep the space open for 24–48 h if cavity is significant.

7. Remove tourniquet; ensure hemostasis; apply non-adherent dressing.

COMPLICATIONS / SIDE EFFECTS

1. Pain flare, bleeding/hematoma, infection progression, nail plate deformity if nail bed injured.
2. Recurrence if drainage inadequate or if nail spicule remains.
3. Rare: anesthetic reaction, digital nerve irritation.

AFTERCARE & MONITORING

1. Warm water or saline soaks 2–3× daily for 3–5 days; keep dressing clean and dry between soaks.
2. Remove wick after 24–48 h if placed; continue local care until healed.
3. Analgesia: acetaminophen/NSAIDs if appropriate.
4. Antibiotics **only** if cellulitis, lymphangitis, systemic illness, immunocompromise, or oral inoculation (thumb-sucking, nail-biting). Select agents per local guidance.
5. Red flags: worsening pain, spreading erythema, fever, numbness — return promptly.

DISPOSITION

1. Discharge with written care instructions and follow-up in 2–3 days for reassessment.
2. Advise nail-care measures: avoid trauma, trim straight across, avoid biting/picking; consider protective gloves at work.

REFERENCES

NHS — Paronychia (nail fold infection): overview and treatment. https://www.nhs.uk

DermNet NZ — Paronychia: causes and management. https://dermnetnz.org

MyHealth.Alberta.ca — Paronychia: care instructions. https://myhealth.alberta.ca

HealthLink BC — Nail infections and wound care (patient info). https://www.healthlinkbc.ca

British Association of Dermatologists — Patient leaflet: Paronychia. https://www.bad.org.uk

SUBUNGUAL HEMATOMA — TREPHINATION

INDICATIONS

1. Acute, painful subungual hematoma causing significant pressure after crush/impact injury (finger or toe).
2. Intact nail plate adherent to nail bed with no obvious nail-edge laceration or avulsion requiring repair.
3. Short interval from injury (typically within 24–48 hours) and patient seeking rapid pain relief.

CONTRAINDICATIONS / CAUTIONS

1. Clinical signs of nail-bed laceration needing repair (nail plate disruption, edge lifted/avulsed, split nail).
2. Displaced distal phalanx fracture or gross nail deformity—consider imaging and surgical assessment.
3. Overlying cellulitis or suspected digital infection (treat first).

4. Acrylic/gel nails—avoid heat/electrocautery (flammable); use needle technique or consider nail removal if necessary.

5. Relative: coagulopathy/anticoagulation (apply firm hemostasis), delayed presentation with minimal pain.

CONSENT

1. Purpose: decompress hematoma to relieve pain and preserve nail plate.

2. Benefits: rapid pain relief, simple office procedure.

3. Risks: bleeding, infection, transient pain, residual hematoma, nail deformity if matrix injured, thermal injury if heat used, rare injury to nail bed.

4. Alternatives: observation/analgesia if mild, nail-plate removal and nail-bed repair when laceration present.

PREPARATION

1. Consider X-ray if high-energy crush, marked tenderness of distal phalanx, or deformity; a non-displaced fracture does not preclude trephination if nail margins are intact.

2. Asepsis: cleanse digit with chlorhexidine or povidone-iodine; wear gloves; place small sterile drape.

3. Anesthesia often unnecessary; if required,

perform a small intradermal bleb or digital block with 1% lidocaine (no epinephrine per local protocol).

4. Avoid alcohol-based prep drying on the nail if using thermal method (fire risk).

EQUIPMENT

1. Antiseptic swabs, gauze, small sterile drape, gloves.
2. Electrocautery pen **or** 18-gauge needle (or 20G for small nails).
3. Adhesive bandage; optional neutral splint if fracture present.

PROCEDURE — THERMAL TREPHINATION (NOT FOR ACRYLIC NAILS)

1. Identify the darkest central area of the hematoma, avoiding the lunula and proximal nail fold.
2. Touch the electrocautery tip lightly to the nail plate with minimal pressure; allow it to melt through until blood wells up.
3. Permit drainage; gently milk blood from proximal to distal. Enlarge the hole slightly if needed for ongoing drainage.
4. Do not advance the tip once drainage begins to avoid nail-bed burn.

PROCEDURE — NEEDLE "DRILL" TREPHINATION

1. Place the bevel of an 18G needle perpendicular to the nail over the darkest area.
2. Rotate/twist with gentle downward pressure until sudden loss of resistance and blood drainage occur.
3. Allow free drainage; a second hole may be placed if needed. Wipe clean and reassess pain.

COMPLICATIONS / SIDE EFFECTS

1. Infection, persistent bleeding, residual hematoma, pain flare.
2. Nail deformity or loss (usually from the original injury or if nail bed is damaged).
3. Thermal injury to nail bed (avoid by stopping once drainage starts).

AFTERCARE & MONITORING

1. Cover with clean dressing; change daily for 48–72 h. Short warm soaks may aid drainage after 24 h.
2. Analgesia as needed. Avoid tight footwear or further trauma.
3. Antibiotics are **not** routinely indicated; consider only if open wounds/contamination or cellulitis per local guidance.
4. Return precautions: increasing pain, redness, warmth, fever, pus, or persistent throbbing.

5. If radiograph shows a significant fracture or nail-bed laceration is suspected, arrange hand/ orthopedic follow-up.

DISPOSITION

1. Discharge with written care instructions and follow-up as needed (2–3 days if symptoms persist).

REFERENCES

Royal Children's Hospital (Melbourne) — Clinical Practice Guidelines: Fingertip and nail injuries. https://www.rch.org.au

MyHealth.Alberta.ca — Subungual Hematoma: Care Instructions. https://myhealth.alberta.ca

Healthdirect Australia — Subungual haematoma. https://www.healthdirect.gov.au

AAOS OrthoInfo — Fingertip Injuries and Amputations (patient information). https://orthoinfo. aaos.org

HealthLink BC — Hand and finger injuries: care. https://www.healthlinkbc.ca

FELON (PULP SPACE) — INCISION & DRAINAGE (I&D)

INDICATIONS

1. Severe throbbing pain, tense swelling, and tenderness of the distal pulp space (finger/thumb) with fluctuance.
2. Failure of early conservative measures (elevation, warm soaks, antibiotics when indicated).
3. Suspicion of abscess compartmentalized within digital pulp (often post puncture/penetrating injury).

CONTRAINDICATIONS / SPECIAL CONSIDERATIONS

1. Suspected **flexor tenosynovitis** (Kanavel signs) — requires urgent hand/surgical consultation.
2. Extensive cellulitis, systemic illness, or immunocompromise — consider IV therapy and specialist input.
3. Children or patients unable to cooperate —

consider procedural sedation/anesthesia if
available.

CONSENT

1. Purpose: decompress and drain the pulp space to
   relieve pain and prevent complications (necrosis,
   osteomyelitis).
2. Benefits: rapid symptom relief and reduced risk of
   tissue loss.
3. Risks: bleeding, infection spread, digital nerve/
   artery injury, nail bed injury, painful scar,
   recurrence; rare osteomyelitis.
4. Alternatives: continued conservative care
   only in very early cellulitic phase without abscess;
   otherwise not adequate.

PREPARATION

1. Assess for foreign body and distal phalanx
   fracture — consider X-ray if penetrating trauma or
   bony tenderness.
2. Check tetanus status. Mark incision site; avoid
   volar transverse or 'fish-mouth' incisions (risk
   ischemic flap).
3. Asepsis: chlorhexidine or povidone-iodine; sterile
   gloves and small drape.
4. Digital nerve block with 1% lidocaine (no
   epinephrine per local protocol); apply a digital
   tourniquet (penrose) for a dry field.

EQUIPMENT

1. Antiseptic swabs, sterile gloves, gauze, small sterile drape, adhesive dressing.

2. Syringe (5–10 mL) with 25–27G needle; 1% lidocaine.

3. No. 11 blade; small hemostat; blunt elevator/freer; fine forceps.

4. Irrigation (saline); small wick/ribbon gauze; optional splint for comfort.

5. Culture swab if unusual exposure (bites, water) or severe infection; antibiotics per local guidance when indicated.

PROCEDURE STEPS — LATERAL LONGITUDINAL INCISION

1. Select the **lateral** aspect of the distal pulp, just **ulnar side** for index/middle and **radial side** for ring/little fingers to avoid most sensitive contact surfaces; stay distal to the DIP flexion crease.

2. Make a small **longitudinal** incision over the point of maximal fluctuance, parallel to the nail plate; avoid crossing midline and avoid transverse volar incisions.

3. Gently spread with a hemostat to break septations within the pulp compartments; avoid aggressive curettage to protect neurovascular bundles.

4. Express pus and irrigate copiously with warm saline until clear.

5. Place a small wick to prevent premature closure for 24–48 h if cavity significant. Remove tourniquet; ensure hemostasis; apply non-adherent dressing.

COMPLICATIONS / SIDE EFFECTS

1. Persistent infection or recurrence, osteomyelitis of distal phalanx, painful scar or sensory changes.

2. Digital artery/nerve injury (avoid deep dissection near midline), nail bed injury if incision too dorsal.

3. Stiffness; consider early gentle range of motion after acute pain subsides.

AFTERCARE & MONITORING

1. Elevate hand; warm soaks 2–3× daily; change dressing after each soak for 3–5 days.

2. Analgesia as needed. If cellulitis or systemic signs present, prescribe antibiotics targeting staphylococci/streptococci per local guidance.

3. Return precautions: worsening pain, spreading erythema, fever, numbness, purulent drainage, or failure to improve in 24–48 h.

4. Consider splinting in a functional position for comfort for 24–48 h; begin gentle motion thereafter.

DISPOSITION

1. Discharge with written instructions and follow-up in 24–48 h for wick removal and reassessment.
2. Urgent specialist review if tendon sheath involvement suspected, osteomyelitis concern, or atypical organisms.

REFERENCES

American Family Physician — Acute Hand Infections (open access). https://www.aafp.org

Royal Children's Hospital (Melbourne) — Clinical Practice Guidelines: Cellulitis and skin infections / fingertip injuries (open access). https://www.rch.org.au

MyHealth.Alberta.ca — Hand infection care instructions. https://myhealth.alberta.ca

HealthLink BC — Hand and finger infections: care. https://www.healthlinkbc.ca

AAOS OrthoInfo — Fingertip Injuries and Infections (patient information). https://orthoinfo.aaos.org

WOUND CLOSURE

SUTURING & STAPLING OF LACERATIONS

INDICATIONS

1. Simple, clean lacerations requiring primary closure for hemostasis, function, or cosmesis.
2. Selected contaminated wounds after irrigation/ debridement; consider delayed primary closure if high-risk.
3. Stapling: straight linear wounds on scalp/trunk/ extremities where cosmesis is less critical and hair is present (scalp).

CONTRAINDICATIONS / CAUTIONS

1. Bites (human/animal), grossly contaminated/ crush injuries—consider delayed closure and antibiotics per local guidance.
2. Deep structure injury (nerve/tendon/duct/artery), open fracture, or foreign body not removed— consult/transfer.
3. Through-and-through oral/cheek wounds, eyelid margin, vermilion border alignment—specialist

techniques.

4. Relative: delayed presentation with devitalized edges, immunocompromise, poorly perfused tissue.

CONSENT

1. Purpose: align wound edges to promote healing and function/cosmesis.

2. Benefits: faster healing, reduced infection risk (if cleaned), improved appearance.

3. Risks: infection, dehiscence, scar/keloid, hematoma, pain/numbness, need for suture removal, allergic reaction to materials.

4. Alternatives: tissue adhesive/steri-strips, secondary intention, delayed primary closure.

PREPARATION

1. Hemostasis (direct pressure; judicious epinephrine with local protocol).

2. Analgesia/anesthesia: local infiltration or field block with 1% lidocaine ± epinephrine; digital block for fingers/toes per protocol.

3. Irrigation: pressurized saline (aim ~5–8 psi) using 35–50 mL syringe + 18–19G catheter; typical **50–100 mL per cm** of wound.

4. Explore full depth; remove foreign material; conservative debridement of devitalized tissue.

5. Tetanus assessment and prophylaxis per

CDC; antibiotics only if indicated (bites, gross contamination, through-and-through oral, immunocompromise).

EQUIPMENT

1. Sterile gloves, drapes; wound irrigation set (syringe + angiocatheter), saline.

2. Instruments: forceps (toothed for skin), needle driver, scissors; stapler & remover if stapling.

3. Suture: monofilament nylon/polypropylene for skin (e.g., **face 5-0/6-0; scalp 3-0/4-0 or staples; trunk 3-0/4-0; limb 4-0; hand 5-0; foot 4-0**).

4. Deep dermal (absorbable 3-0/4-0) if under tension; adhesive strips/tissue adhesive for low-tension linear wounds.

PROCEDURE — SUTURING (SIMPLE INTERRUPTED/DEEP DERMAL + SKIN)

1. Prep and drape. Anesthetize and irrigate thoroughly; achieve hemostasis.

2. Assess for layered closure: place **deep dermal absorbable** sutures to reduce tension when depth >5 mm or gaping.

3. Place **simple interrupted** skin stitches 3–5 mm from edge, spaced 5–10 mm; evert wound edges. Adjust spacing on face (closer, finer).

4. Align landmarks (vermilion border first stitch; brow margins).

5. Alternative patterns: vertical mattress for eversion in thick skin; horizontal mattress for fragile skin; running locked for hemostasis (avoid if contamination).

PROCEDURE — STAPLING (SCALP/ TRUNK)

1. Approximate edges with forceps; place staples 5–10 mm apart perpendicular to wound; ensure eversion.
2. Avoid face, hands, or joints where contour/ cosmesis critical. Use staple remover for atraumatic removal.

SPECIAL SITUATIONS (BRIEF)

1. Face: irrigate well; **avoid shaving eyebrows**; prefer 5-0/6-0 nylon; remove in **5–7 days**.
2. Scalp: consider staples or 3-0/4-0 nylon; remove in **7–10 days**; hair-apposition technique is an option for low-tension.
3. Lips: align vermilion first with **6-0** nylon; consider absorbable mucosal sutures.
4. Hands/Feet/Joints: assess tendon/nerve; splint if over joint; remove in **10–14 days**.
5. High-risk wounds (bites, farm injuries): debride, irrigate copiously, consider delayed primary closure and antibiotics.

COMPLICATIONS / SIDE EFFECTS

1. Infection, dehiscence, hematoma/seroma, hypertrophic/keloid scar, suture track marks.
2. Missed tendon/nerve injury, retained foreign body, allergic/contact dermatitis from adhesives/tape.

AFTERCARE & MONITORING

1. Keep dry for 24–48 h, then daily gentle cleanse; apply petrolatum (preferred over topical antibiotics unless indicated).
2. Elevation/immobilization for limbs and joints; dressing changes if soiled.
3. Suture removal timing (typical): **face 5–7 d; scalp 7–10 d; trunk 10–14 d; upper limb 10–14 d; lower limb 12–14 d; hand/foot 10–14 d**.
4. Sun protection; consider silicone gel/sheets after epithelialization for scar modulation.
5. Return if increasing pain, redness, warmth, purulent drainage, fever, numbness, or wound separation.

DISPOSITION

1. Provide tetanus documentation and wound care sheet; plan removal appointment per site.
2. Arrange specialist referral if complex injury, suspected deep structure damage, or poor perfusion.

REFERENCES

American Family Physician — Laceration Repair: A Practical Approach (open access). https://www. aafp.org

Centers for Disease Control and Prevention (CDC) — Tetanus Prophylaxis for Wound Management. https://www.cdc.gov

NHS — Cuts and lacerations: treatment and self-care. https://www.nhs.uk

Healthdirect Australia — Cuts, grazes and lacerations. https://www.healthdirect.gov.au

MyHealth.Alberta.ca — Stitches and staples: care instructions. https://myhealth.alberta.ca

TISSUE ADHESIVE (CYANOACRYLATE) — WOUND CLOSURE

INDICATIONS

1. Simple, clean, linear lacerations with well-approximated, low-tension edges (typically <5 cm).
2. Face, scalp (adjunct to hair apposition), trunk, and some extremity wounds where immobilization is feasible.
3. Alternative to sutures for needle-averse patients or pediatric closures.

CONTRAINDICATIONS / CAUTIONS

1. Contaminated, crush, bite or puncture wounds; devitalized edges; active bleeding not controlled.
2. High-tension sites (joints, hands/feet over movement areas) unless immobilized; mucosal or moist intertriginous areas.
3. Allergy to cyanoacrylates; proximity to eyes without eye protection; deep wounds needing layered closure.

CONSENT

1. Purpose: close superficial skin edges without needles.
2. Benefits: quick application, no removal visit, comparable cosmetic outcome to sutures in low-tension wounds.
3. Risks: wound dehiscence (higher vs. sutures in high-tension areas), contact dermatitis, heat/sting, accidental adhesion to unintended tissues, foreign-body reaction (rare).
4. Alternatives: sutures, staples (location dependent), adhesive strips, delayed primary closure.

PREPARATION

1. Achieve hemostasis and irrigate thoroughly; debride as needed.
2. Dry skin edges completely; protect surrounding skin and eyes (use petroleum/ophthalmic ointment barrier if near eye).
3. Approximate edges precisely with forceps or finger pressure.

EQUIPMENT

1. Tissue adhesive (e.g., 2-octyl or n-butyl cyanoacrylate single-use ampoule).
2. Gauze, forceps, optional skin barrier (petrolatum), and protective drapes.

3. Optional: steri-strips for reinforcement; splint for high-mobility areas.

PROCEDURE — APPLICATION

1. With edges pinched together and dry, paint a **thin layer** of adhesive **across** (not into) the approximated epidermal edges; avoid adhesive within the wound.
2. Allow ~30 seconds to polymerize; apply 2–3 thin layers, letting each dry before the next.
3. Release traction once firm. If seepage into the wound occurs, allow to dry—do not wipe into the wound.
4. If near the eye, place gauze to shield; immediately irrigate with saline if adhesive contacts the eye and seek ophthalmology advice.

COMPLICATIONS / SIDE EFFECTS

1. Dehiscence if used on high-tension/motion areas; adhesive dermatitis or blistering.
2. Accidental adhesion to gloves/adjacent skin; thermal sensation on application.
3. Infection risk similar to sutures when wound properly prepared.

AFTERCARE & MONITORING

1. Keep dry for 24 hours; brief showers thereafter; avoid ointments over adhesive (may loosen).

2. Adhesive typically sloughs in 5–10 days; do not pick. Avoid sun/soaking; immobilize area if over a joint.

3. Return if increasing pain, redness, warmth, purulent drainage, or wound separation.

DISPOSITION

1. No removal needed; arrange follow-up PRN or within 5–7 days for cosmetic check in high-visibility areas.

REFERENCES

American Family Physician — Using Tissue Adhesive for Wound Repair (open access). https://www.aafp.org

Royal Children's Hospital (Melbourne) — Clinical Practice Guidelines: Lacerations (open access). https://www.rch.org.au

NHS — Cuts and lacerations: treatment and self-care. https://www.nhs.uk

Healthdirect Australia — Cuts, grazes and lacerations. https://www.healthdirect.gov.au

MyHealth.Alberta.ca — Stitches, staples, and skin adhesive: care instructions. https://myhealth.alberta.ca

ADHESIVE STRIPS (STERI-STRIPS) — WOUND CLOSURE

INDICATIONS

1. Superficial, clean, straight lacerations with minimal tension and well-approximated edges.
2. Fragile/atrophic skin where sutures risk tearing; after suture removal to support wound.
3. Adjunct over sutures or tissue adhesive to reduce tension.

CONTRAINDICATIONS / CAUTIONS

1. Moist areas (axilla, groin), hair-bearing scalp without preparation, heavily contoured or mobile sites unless reinforced.
2. Contaminated, jagged, crush or bite wounds; actively bleeding wounds; deep wounds requiring layered closure.

CONSENT

1. Purpose: approximate skin edges non-invasively.
2. Benefits: painless, quick, no anesthesia, minimal

scarring risk.

3. Risks: dehiscence if tension high or strips loosen, contact dermatitis to adhesive, maceration if kept wet.

4. Alternatives: tissue adhesive, sutures, staples, delayed closure.

PREPARATION

1. Irrigate/debride thoroughly; achieve hemostasis.

2. Clip hair if needed; dry skin meticulously. Apply **tincture of benzoin** or adhesive adjunct to improve adherence (avoid if allergic).

3. Cut strips to length before application.

EQUIPMENT

1. Adhesive skin closures (Steri-Strips or equivalent).

2. Tincture of benzoin/adhesive adjunct (optional), gauze, scissors, forceps.

3. Reinforcement: additional strips laid perpendicular across ends; cover dressing.

PROCEDURE — APPLICATION

1. Align wound edges with fingers/forceps; starting at the **center**, place first strip perpendicular to the wound to achieve edge eversion.

2. Add additional strips spaced 2–3 mm apart

toward the wound ends; avoid bridging moisture or tension gaps.

3. Place a few **parallel reinforcing strips** along the wound axis to secure perpendicular strips, especially in mobile areas.

4. If combination with tissue adhesive: apply strips **after** adhesive cures, not before.

COMPLICATIONS / SIDE EFFECTS

1. Edge maceration if left wet; premature loosening; contact dermatitis; wound separation if tension underestimated.

AFTERCARE & MONITORING

1. Keep dry for 24–48 hours; then brief showers allowed. Pat dry; do not soak.

2. Strips usually loosen and fall off in 5–10 days; trim loose ends rather than peel.

3. Return if worsening pain, redness, discharge, or if wound gaps open.

DISPOSITION

1. No removal required; advise protective dressing for friction areas for several days.

REFERENCES

Royal Children's Hospital (Melbourne) — Clinical Practice Guidelines: Lacerations (open access). https://www.rch.org.au

NHS — Cuts and lacerations: treatment and self-care. https://www.nhs.uk

Healthdirect Australia — Cuts, grazes and lacerations. https://www.healthdirect.gov.au

MyHealth.Alberta.ca — Stitches, staples, and skin adhesive: care instructions. https://myhealth.alberta.ca

American Family Physician — Essentials of Skin Laceration Repair (open access). https://www.aafp.org

ENT / EYE

EPISTAXIS — ANTERIOR NASAL PACKING

INDICATIONS

1. Persistent anterior epistaxis after 10–15 minutes of firm compression and topical vasoconstrictor.
2. Diffuse oozing from Kiesselbach's plexus or when cautery is not possible/unsuccessful.
3. Anticoagulated or fragile mucosa where tamponade is preferred to cautery.

CONTRAINDICATIONS / CAUTIONS

1. Suspected posterior epistaxis (bleeding from both nares/oropharynx, older patient, heavy bleeding) — consider ENT and posterior control.
2. Midface/cribriform or basilar skull fracture, significant facial trauma — avoid nasal instrumentation.
3. Airway compromise, hemodynamic instability — resuscitate and involve ENT/anesthesia.
4. Coagulopathy/anticoagulation — correct/ reverse when appropriate; use gentle technique.

CONSENT

1. Purpose: tamponade anterior bleeding to achieve hemostasis.
2. Benefits: rapid control, avoids operative intervention in many cases.
3. Risks: pain/pressure, mucosal injury, infection/ sinusitis, otitis media, rare toxic shock syndrome, rebleed on removal.
4. Alternatives: ongoing compression/topical therapy, chemical/electrocautery if focal source, posterior packing/ENT procedures if indicated.

PREPARATION

1. PPE for splash risk; seated position with patient leaning forward; suction ready.
2. Ask patient to blow out clots. Apply topical vasoconstrictor/anesthetic (e.g., oxymetazoline + 2–4% lidocaine) on pledgets for 10 minutes.
3. Consider topical tranexamic acid (e.g., 500 mg/5 mL on pledgets) before packing.
4. Identify focal bleeding under suction; if discrete and accessible, attempt **single-side silver nitrate cautery** (avoid bilateral septal cautery) before packing.

EQUIPMENT

1. Light/headlamp, nasal speculum, bayonet forceps, Yankauer/Frazier suction.

2. Topical vasoconstrictor (e.g., oxymetazoline/ phenylephrine), topical/local anesthetic, optional tranexamic acid.

3. Packing options: **Non-absorbable** (Merocel®/ PVA nasal tampon; ribbon gauze), **Balloon device** (e.g., Rapid Rhino®), **Absorbable** (gelatin sponge/oxidized cellulose).

4. Syringe with sterile water (to lubricate/activate PVA or balloon), scissors, external moustache dressing.

PROCEDURE STEPS — QUICK ALGORITHM

1. 1) Compress + vasoconstrictor pledgets 10 minutes → reassess.

2. 2) If focal source seen → **cauterize** (single side).

3. 3) If still bleeding or diffuse → **pack** using one of the following methods.

PACKING TECHNIQUE — PVA NASAL TAMPON (MEROCEL®)

1. Moisten tampon tip with sterile water or anesthetic solution (avoid petroleum).

2. Insert **horizontally along the floor** of the nasal cavity to full length until just posterior to vestibule; avoid upward angulation.

3. Instill a few mL sterile water to expand. Place

external dressing. Confirm hemostasis; repeat in contralateral nostril only if needed.

PACKING TECHNIQUE — RIBBON GAUZE

1. Soak 1–1.25 cm ribbon gauze in petrolatum or antibiotic ointment.
2. Using bayonet forceps and speculum, **layer from posterior to anterior** in accordion fashion, filling the nasal cavity without excessive pressure.
3. Leave a small tail externally and apply external dressing.

PACKING TECHNIQUE — BALLOON DEVICE (E.G., RAPID RHINO®)

1. Soak the device in sterile water to activate surface. Insert horizontally along the floor until the marker aligns with the ala.
2. Inflate balloon **gradually with air** (typical 4–10 mL depending on size) until hemostasis and patient comfort; do not over-inflate.
3. Secure device; apply moustache dressing.

ABSORBABLE PACKING (WHEN MINIMAL/MODERATE BLEEDING OR ANTICOAGULATED)

1. Place gelatin sponge or oxidized cellulose over the anterior septum/bleed and compress gently. No removal required; it dissolves.

MONITORING, REMOVAL & AFTERCARE

1. Observe 30–60 minutes to ensure hemostasis; check vitals, oxygen if needed.

2. Typical duration in situ: **24–48 hours** (absorbables do not require removal). **Moisten PVA** with saline before removal to reduce trauma; fully deflate balloons before withdrawal.

3. Antibiotics: **not routinely required** for simple anterior packing; consider only if immunocompromised, valvular heart disease, purulent sinusitis, or packing >48 h per local guidance.

4. Discharge instructions: avoid nose blowing, heavy lifting, hot drinks/alcohol for 48–72 h; sneeze with mouth open; humidify air; apply petrolatum to anterior septum; use saline sprays after pack removal.

5. Return urgently for persistent bleeding, fever >38 °C, foul discharge, severe pain, or breathing difficulty. Arrange **ENT/primary care follow-up in 24–48 h**.

DISPOSITION

1. Discharge if stable and controlled; admit if posterior bleed suspected, significant comorbidity/anticoagulation with large bleed, hypoxia, or social concerns.

REFERENCES

NICE CKS — Epistaxis (open access). https://cks.nice.org.uk

ENT UK — First aid and management for nosebleeds (patient info). https://www.entuk.org

Royal Children's Hospital (Melbourne) — Clinical Practice Guideline: Epistaxis. https://www.rch.org.au

Emergency Care BC — Epistaxis Clinical Summary. https://emergencycarebc.ca

American Family Physician — Epistaxis: Outpatient Management (open access). https://www.aafp.org

NHS — Nosebleed: treatment and self-care. https://www.nhs.uk

PERITONSILLAR ABSCESS — NEEDLE ASPIRATION

INDICATIONS

1. Suspected peritonsillar abscess with trismus, muffled "hot-potato" voice, unilateral peritonsillar swelling, uvular deviation, severe odynophagia/ drooling.
2. Failure of initial medical management or significant airway/analgesia needs requiring decompression.
3. Diagnostic confirmation when peritonsillar cellulitis vs. abscess is uncertain.

CONTRAINDICATIONS / CAUTIONS

1. Airway compromise or inability to protect airway — manage airway and obtain urgent ENT/ anesthesia support first.
2. Uncooperative patient without ability to provide adequate anesthesia/sedation.
3. Coagulopathy/anticoagulation (optimize and use meticulous hemostasis).

4. Suspicion of deep neck space infection beyond peritonsillar area (parapharyngeal/ retropharyngeal) — consider imaging/ENT consult.

5. Children or severe trismus: consider ENT involvement or procedural sedation.

CONSENT

1. Purpose: evacuate pus to relieve pain and improve swallowing; obtain sample for culture if indicated.

2. Benefits: rapid symptom relief, diagnostic clarity, may avoid operative drainage.

3. Risks: bleeding, aspiration of pus/blood, airway spasm, dental/lip trauma, carotid puncture (rare), recurrence or need for further drainage.

4. Alternatives: continued IV/PO antibiotics and observation if cellulitis only; incision & drainage; operative drainage/tonsillectomy per ENT.

PREPARATION

1. Monitoring: IV access, suction ready; position seated, slightly leaning forward; good lighting/ headlamp.

2. Asepsis and protection: eye/face protection for splatter; use bite block or tongue depressor. Have Yankauer suction and basin ready.

3. Topical anesthesia: lidocaine 2–4% spray or viscous gargle (avoid benzocaine where

methemoglobinemia is a concern).

4. Local anesthesia: 1% lidocaine with or without epinephrine per local protocol; infiltrate mucosa superficially at target site.

5. Needle guard: cap/guard to limit depth to ~10 mm (1 cm) to reduce carotid risk.

EQUIPMENT

1. Tongue depressor or laryngoscope blade, good light/headlamp, bite block.

2. Suction (Yankauer), kidney dish; gauze; PPE (eye/face shield).

3. 10 mL syringe with 18- or 20-gauge needle; needle guard for 1 cm depth.

4. Lidocaine spray/viscous; 1% lidocaine for infiltration; optional epinephrine per local protocol.

5. Specimen container for culture (if indicated).

LANDMARKS & SAFE ZONES

1. Target the **superior pole of the tonsil** at the point of maximal swelling, just **medial to the anterior tonsillar pillar** and **superior to the tonsil**.

2. Avoid the **posterolateral** area beyond the posterior pillar where the carotid artery lies ~2–2.5 cm posterior-lateral — hence the 1 cm needle guard.

3. If no pus on first pass, adjust slightly and sample

superior, middle, and inferior positions, always with depth limited to 1 cm.

PROCEDURE STEPS — NEEDLE ASPIRATION

1. Dry mucosa; apply topical anesthetic. Infiltrate small amount of local at target.
2. Place needle guard ($\approx$10 mm exposed). Aspirate at the superior pole first while directing **medially** toward the tonsillar fossa; apply gentle suction.
3. If pus returns, continue aspiration until cavity decompresses. Suction pooled secretions to prevent aspiration.
4. If no pus, repeat limited passes at middle and inferior points over the fluctuance, maintaining 1 cm depth limit.
5. If aspiration unsuccessful but suspicion remains high, consider small stab incision and blunt opening **only in a controlled setting** or obtain ENT assistance.
6. Send aspirate for Gram stain/culture if indicated (recurrent, immunocompromised, atypical). Achieve hemostasis with pressure/ vasoconstrictor-soaked swab.

COMPLICATIONS / SIDE EFFECTS

1. Bleeding, vasovagal event, aspiration of pus/

blood, airway compromise.

2. Inadequate drainage/recurrence; extension to deeper spaces (rare with adequate management).

3. Very rare: carotid injury (mitigated by 1 cm depth guard and medial approach).

AFTERCARE & MEDICAL MANAGEMENT

1. Observe for **30–60 minutes** for bleeding and airway tolerance of oral intake.

2. Antibiotics (examples per local guidance): amoxicillin-clavulanate or clindamycin (if penicillin-allergic). Tailor to culture if obtained.

3. Analgesia and hydration; consider a single dose **dexamethasone** to reduce pain/edema (per local protocol).

4. Advise soft diet, saltwater rinses; strict return precautions for bleeding, dyspnea, or worsening pain/swelling.

5. Follow-up with ENT or primary care within **24–48 h**; earlier if symptoms recur or worsen.

DISPOSITION

1. Discharge if tolerating PO and pain controlled; admit if airway risk, dehydration, sepsis, significant comorbidities, or inadequate home support.

REFERENCES

NHS — Quinsy (peritonsillar abscess): overview and treatment. https://www.nhs.uk

NICE CKS — Sore throat (acute): assessment and complications including peritonsillar abscess (open access). https://cks.nice.org.uk

ENT UK — Patient information: Quinsy (Peritonsillar Abscess). https://www.entuk.org

Healthdirect Australia — Quinsy (peritonsillar abscess). https://www.healthdirect.gov.au

American Family Physician — Peritonsillar Abscess (open access review). https://www.aafp.org

EAR CANAL IRRIGATION & CERUMEN REMOVAL

INDICATIONS

1. Symptomatic cerumen impaction causing hearing loss, fullness, pain, tinnitus, cough (Arnold's reflex), or vertigo.
2. Obstructed view of tympanic membrane (e.g., to assess infection, perforation, or fit hearing aids).

CONTRAINDICATIONS / CAUTIONS

1. Known or suspected **tympanic membrane perforation**, presence of **tympanostomy tubes**, or **post-mastoid/ear surgery** (unless ENT-directed).
2. Active otitis externa or severe otalgia; **unilateral deafness** (irrigate the better ear only with extreme caution or avoid).
3. Canal stenosis/exostoses where irrigation may trap fluid; impacted foreign body (especially hygroscopic objects).
4. Relative: anticoagulation/coagulopathy (risk

canal bleeding/hematoma), immunocompromise/ diabetes (higher otitis externa risk).

CONSENT

1. Purpose: remove obstructive earwax to relieve symptoms and allow examination.
2. Benefits: improved hearing/comfort, visualization of TM.
3. Risks: pain, canal abrasion/bleeding, otitis externa, vertigo (from cold/warm water), tinnitus, **TM perforation** (rare).
4. Alternatives: cerumenolytic drops alone, **manual curettage/microsuction**, ENT referral.

PREPARATION

1. Confirm indication with otoscopy; if TM cannot be seen and perforation suspected, **do not irrigate** — consider microsuction/ENT.
2. Pre-soften: carbamide peroxide, mineral/olive oil, or sodium bicarbonate drops **15–30 min** pre-procedure (or 3–5 days at home).
3. Use **body-temperature water ($\approx$37 °C)** to prevent caloric vertigo; set up good lighting/ suction; provide splash protection.

EQUIPMENT

1. Otoscope with specula; basin/shoulder drape; towels; PPE/eye shield.

2. 20–60 mL syringe with **soft catheter tip** (e.g., 16–18G IV cannula sheath without needle) or bulb syringe; irrigation bottle system if available.

3. Warm sterile/clean tap water or saline; cerumenolytic drops; curette/Jobson Horne loop for residual wax; suction if available.

PROCEDURE — IRRIGATION

1. Seat patient upright, head tilted toward the side being treated; place basin beneath ear.

2. Straighten canal (adult: pinna up/back; child: down/back).

3. Aim the stream **superior-posterior canal wall**, not directly at the TM; deliver short, gentle pulses while observing patient comfort.

4. Allow return flow into basin; reassess with otoscope after each 30–60 mL. Repeat as needed.

5. Stop if severe pain, vertigo, nausea, or bleeding. Dry canal afterwards (gently wick with gauze tip); consider a few drops of acetic acid 2% or isopropyl alcohol-based drying drops if not contraindicated by TM status and local guidance.

PROCEDURE — MANUAL REMOVAL (WHEN IRRIGATION UNSUITABLE)

1. Under direct visualization, use curette/loop or microsuction to remove softened wax in small pieces.

2. Avoid deep blind curettage; stop if poor visualization or patient discomfort — consider ENT referral.

COMPLICATIONS / SIDE EFFECTS

1. Canal abrasion/bleed, otitis externa, transient dizziness, tinnitus, cough reflex, TM perforation (rare).

2. Incomplete removal requiring repeat session or alternative method.

AFTERCARE & MONITORING

1. Advise **ear-drying precautions** for 24–48 h; avoid cotton buds/Q-tips.

2. If canal abraded or high risk for otitis externa, consider prophylactic **acetic acid 2%** drops per local protocol; otherwise not routinely required.

3. Return if pain, discharge, fever, or hearing does not improve; consider audiology/ENT if recurrent impaction.

4. Preventive tips: periodic softening drops for recurrent wax, avoid objects in ear, manage hearing aids per manufacturer guidance.

DISPOSITION

1. Document method, side, volume used, patient tolerance, and TM appearance post-procedure; arrange follow-up PRN.

REFERENCES

NICE CKS — Earwax (open access). https://cks.nice.org.uk

NHS — Earwax build-up: treatment and self-care. https://www.nhs.uk

American Academy of Otolaryngology–Head and Neck Surgery (AAO-HNS) — Earwax (Cerumen) patient information. https://www.enthealth.org

Healthdirect Australia — Earwax (cerumen). https://www.healthdirect.gov.au

MyHealth.Alberta.ca — Earwax blockage: care instructions. https://myhealth.alberta.ca

Royal Children's Hospital (Melbourne) — Clinical Guidelines: Ear conditions (relevant ear toileting/irrigation cautions). https://www.rch.org.au

GENERAL SURGICAL/ED INFECTIONS

REMOVAL OF FOREIGN BODIES —
SKIN, EYE, EAR, NOSE, SOFT TISSUE

INDICATIONS

1. Symptomatic or potentially harmful foreign body (pain, infection risk, obstruction, vision/hearing compromise).
2. Diagnostic clarification when retained material suspected (history of penetrating injury or unilateral discharge).

CONTRAINDICATIONS / RED FLAGS (REFER/URGENT CARE)

1. Airway compromise, button battery/magnet ingestion or in ear/nose, suspected globe rupture or high-velocity eye injury.
2. Deep soft-tissue FB near neurovascular structures/tendons, penetrating neck/torso injuries.
3. Uncooperative child without safe restraint/ sedation; lack of appropriate equipment/lighting.

CONSENT & PREP

1. Explain purpose, benefits, risks (pain, bleeding, infection, incomplete removal). Obtain consent.
2. Analgesia/anesthesia as appropriate (topical, local infiltration, digital block). PPE, good lighting, suction ready.
3. Assess tetanus status; irrigate/clean field; consider imaging (X-ray for radiopaque; ultrasound for radiolucent/organic).

SKIN (SUPERFICIAL) & SOFT TISSUE

1. Superficial splinters/thorns: cleanse; grasp with fine forceps; if embedded, make a small tangential incision after local anesthesia; remove along entry path.
2. Glass/metal: irrigate copiously; consider X-ray to detect fragments; avoid blind probing.
3. Organic (wood/plant): higher infection risk — remove fully; consider ultrasound localization for radiolucent pieces.
4. Soft-tissue FB: small incision directly over palpable tip; use blunt dissection with hemostat; avoid neurovascular injury; stop if not easily retrievable and arrange imaging/referral.
5. Aftercare: irrigate; consider antibiotics only if contaminated bite/farm wounds or plantar puncture per local guidance; update tetanus; dressing and return precautions.

EYE (CORNEAL/CONJUNCTIVAL) — SUPERFICIAL ONLY

1. Red flags: globe rupture (teardrop pupil, decreased vision, positive Seidel), high-velocity metal (risk intraocular FB), large central corneal defects — shield and urgent ophthalmology.

2. Technique: topical anesthetic; fluorescein stain; evert upper lid to check for tarsal FB.

3. Removal: moistened cotton swab to sweep away superficial FB away from central visual axis; if adherent peripheral FB, use 25-27G needle under magnification/slit lamp to gently lift edge; avoid central cornea if not confident.

4. Rust ring (metal): partial removal may be attempted if trained; otherwise next-day ophthalmology for burr.

5. Aftercare: topical antibiotic ointment/drop for corneal abrasion per local guidance; avoid contact lenses until healed; urgent review if pain/ photophobia persists.

EAR CANAL

1. Red flags: button battery or paired magnets — **urgent removal**; do not delay. Suspected TM perforation: avoid irrigation.

2. Insects: kill first with warm mineral/olive oil or 2% lidocaine, then remove with suction/forceps.

3. Spherical beads/seeds: avoid irrigation if they

swell; use right-angle hook, suction, or curette under direct visualization.

4. Do not use cyanoacrylate in canal. Stop if bleeding, pain, or poor visualization; refer.

5. Aftercare: inspect TM; treat canal abrasions with topical therapy if indicated; safety-net for pain, discharge, fever.

NOSE

1. Red flags: button battery or magnets — **immediate removal**; prevent mucosal necrosis.

2. First-line positive pressure: patient blow; "parent's kiss" (adult seals mouth over child's mouth, occludes opposite nostril, gives sharp puff).

3. If visible: use hook or forceps to sweep object forward along floor of nose; avoid pushing posteriorly; avoid blind probing.

4. Avoid irrigation (aspiration risk; some objects swell).

5. Aftercare: observe for bleeding/aspiration; ENT follow-up if mucosal injury or if multiple attempts unsuccessful.

COMPLICATIONS / SIDE EFFECTS

1. Bleeding, pain, infection, incomplete removal/ retained fragments, tissue injury.

2. Eye: corneal abrasion, ulceration; Ear/Nose:

canal/lateral wall laceration, TM perforation, aspiration of nasal FB.

3. Soft tissue: neurovascular injury, migration, foreign-body granuloma.

AFTERCARE & DISPOSITION

1. Provide wound care instructions; analgesia; antibiotic use based on site and contamination per local guidance.

2. Update tetanus as indicated (clean minor vs. dirty major wounds).

3. Clear return precautions: worsening pain, redness/swelling, fever, purulent discharge, vision/hearing changes, continued unilateral foul-smelling nasal discharge.

4. Arrange specialist follow-up for ocular injuries, canal lacerations/TM perforation, nasal mucosal damage, deep soft-tissue FB, or if initial attempts fail.

REFERENCES

Royal Children's Hospital (Melbourne) — Clinical Practice Guidelines: Foreign bodies in the ear and nose; Eye (corneal foreign body/abrasion). https://www.rch.org.au

ENT UK — Patient information: Objects in the ear and nose. https://www.entuk.org

American Academy of Ophthalmology (EyeSmart) — Corneal foreign body (patient info). https://www.aao.org

NHS — Foreign objects: eye/ear/nose; Splinters. https://www.nhs.uk

Healthdirect Australia — Objects in the ear and nose; Eye injuries; Splinters. https://www.healthdirect.gov.au

Centers for Disease Control and Prevention (CDC) — Tetanus: wound management. https://www.cdc.gov

MyHealth.Alberta.ca — Removing splinters and wound care. https://myhealth.alberta.ca

CUTANEOUS ABSCESS — INCISION & DRAINAGE (I&D)

INDICATIONS

1. Fluctuant, tender cutaneous collection consistent with abscess, often with surrounding cellulitis.
2. Failure of conservative management (warm compresses, antibiotics when indicated).
3. Systemic symptoms or high-risk location requiring prompt source control.

CONTRAINDICATIONS / CAUTIONS

1. Deep/complex locations (perirectal, peritonsillar, facial triangle, hand deep spaces) — consider imaging/specialist.
2. Large abscess in proximity to major vessels/ nerves — consider ultrasound guidance or referral.
3. Overlying necrosis/necrotizing infection, or suspected foreign body — modify approach and consider imaging.
4. Relative: anticoagulation/coagulopathy

(meticulous hemostasis), poorly controlled diabetes/immunosuppression.

CONSENT

1. Purpose: evacuate pus to relieve pain and treat infection.
2. Benefits: rapid symptom relief, reduced recurrence when source controlled.
3. Risks: bleeding, pain, incomplete drainage/ recurrence, scarring, spread of infection, need for repeat procedure; rare nerve injury depending on site.
4. Alternatives: continued conservative care (often inadequate once fluctuance present), antibiotics alone (not sufficient without drainage).

PREPARATION

1. Assess extent; consider ultrasound if diagnosis uncertain or to map loculations; consider tetanus status.
2. Asepsis: prep skin with chlorhexidine or povidone-iodine; sterile gloves and drape.
3. Analgesia/anesthesia: local infiltration with 1% lidocaine; consider field block. Procedural sedation for children or large/very painful abscesses if available.
4. Mark incision along relaxed skin tension lines; plan most dependent drainage path.

EQUIPMENT

1. Antiseptic swabs, sterile gloves/drape, gauze, suction (if available).
2. Scalpel (#11), hemostats, blunt probe/curette, forceps.
3. Irrigation syringe with saline; culture swab if indicated (recurrent, severe, unusual exposure).
4. Packing (plain ribbon gauze) or loop-drain supplies (2 vessel loops or silicone tubing, 2 skin punctures, suture/ties).
5. Dressings: non-adherent pad, absorbent gauze, tape.

PROCEDURE STEPS — SIMPLE I&D

1. Identify point of maximal fluctuance. Anesthetize and prep field.
2. Make a small linear incision over the most fluctuant area along skin lines; avoid crossing creases when possible.
3. Express pus; gently explore cavity with hemostat/ probe to break loculations.
4. Irrigate with saline until effluent runs clear.
5. Packing: **avoid routine packing** for small (<5 cm), uncomplicated abscesses; consider a small wick only if large cavity, pilonidal/axillary/ groin location, or concern for premature closure.
6. Dress with absorbent gauze; outline cellulitis margin if present to monitor spread.

ALTERNATIVE — LOOP DRAIN (USEFUL FOR CHILDREN/AXILLA/GROIN)

1. Create two small stab incisions at the abscess edges (dependent and superior).
2. Break loculations and irrigate. Pass a soft vessel loop through the cavity and out the second incision; tie loosely to maintain drainage.
3. Cover with dressing. Loop typically remains for ~5–7 days, adjusted per drainage/comfort.

COMPLICATIONS / SIDE EFFECTS

1. Bleeding, pain flare, incomplete drainage/recurrence.
2. Cellulitis progression or systemic infection (rare after adequate drainage).
3. Scarring, sinus formation; rare neurovascular injury depending on site.

AFTERCARE & MONITORING

1. Warm compresses/soaks 2–3× daily for 2–3 days; change dressings daily or when saturated.
2. Analgesia as needed. Elevate involved limb when applicable.
3. Antibiotics: consider if extensive cellulitis, systemic signs, immunocompromise, multiple lesions, extremes of age, or failure of I&D alone; choose per local guidance (e.g., MRSA coverage when appropriate).

4. Return/seek care if increasing pain, fever, spreading erythema, persistent drainage >48–72 h, or if packing/loop dislodges early.

5. Follow-up in 24–48 h if packed/looped; otherwise as needed based on symptoms.

DISPOSITION

1. Discharge with written instructions and safety-net advice; plan follow-up for wound check and dressing change.

2. Urgent reassessment if systemic illness, rapidly worsening infection, or concern for deeper involvement.

REFERENCES

Centers for Disease Control and Prevention (CDC) — Skin and Soft Tissue Infections / MRSA guidance. https://www.cdc.gov

Infectious Diseases Society of America (IDSA) — Practice Guidelines for Skin and Soft Tissue Infections (open access). https://www.idsociety.org

NHS — Skin abscess: treatment and self-care. https://www.nhs.uk

Healthdirect Australia — Skin abscess. https://www.healthdirect.gov.au

MyHealth.Alberta.ca — Skin abscess care instructions. https://myhealth.alberta.ca

American Family Physician — Abscess management and packing evidence (open access). https://www.aafp.org

PILONIDAL ABSCESS —
INCISION & DRAINAGE (I&D)

INDICATIONS

1. Fluctuant, tender abscess in the natal cleft/gluteal fold consistent with pilonidal disease.
2. Failure of conservative measures (warm compresses, analgesia) or systemic symptoms.
3. Need for source control prior to definitive surgical management.

CONTRAINDICATIONS / CAUTIONS

1. Extensive cellulitis, necrotizing infection, or systemic toxicity — urgent surgical assessment.
2. Recurrent/complex disease with multiple pits or lateral tracts — consider imaging and early surgical referral.
3. Relative: anticoagulation/coagulopathy, immunosuppression, pregnancy (antibiotic choice considerations).

CONSENT

1. Purpose: evacuate pus and relieve pain; temporary measure with potential need for later definitive surgery (e.g., cleft-lift, pit excision).
2. Benefits: rapid symptom relief and infection control.
3. Risks: bleeding, pain, incomplete drainage/ recurrence, sinus formation, scarring, need for repeat procedure; rare spread of infection.
4. Alternatives: conservative care (often inadequate once fluctuance present), scheduled operative management when acutely infected state has settled.

PREPARATION

1. Assess extent; consider ultrasound if diagnosis uncertain or to map loculations/pockets.
2. Analgesia/anesthesia: local infiltration or field block with 1% lidocaine; consider procedural sedation for large or very painful abscesses.
3. Asepsis: prep skin with chlorhexidine or povidone-iodine; clip visible hair broadly around the cleft (avoid shaving stubble).
4. Position prone or lateral decubitus with buttocks taped apart for exposure; mark most dependent point for drainage.

EQUIPMENT

1. Antiseptic swabs, sterile gloves/drape, gauze; suction if available.

2. Scalpel (#11), hemostats, blunt probe/curette, forceps.

3. Irrigation syringe with saline; culture swab if severe/recurrent/atypical exposure.

4. Packing (plain ribbon gauze) **or** loop-drain supplies (soft vessel loops/silicone tubing, two small punctures, ties/sutures).

5. Absorbent dressings; consider pressure dressing to reduce re-accumulation.

PROCEDURE STEPS — OFF-MIDLINE I&D (STANDARD)

1. Identify point of maximal fluctuance **lateral to the midline** crease (reduces recurrence and wound complications).

2. Infiltrate anesthetic; make a 1–2 cm **vertical or oblique off-midline incision**; avoid midline horizontal cuts.

3. Express pus; gently explore cavity with hemostat/probe to break septations; remove hair and debris within the cavity.

4. Irrigate thoroughly with warm saline until effluent clears.

5. Packing: avoid routine tight packing. Place a **small wick** only if cavity is large or risk of

premature closure; alternatively use a **loop drain** to maintain dependent drainage.

6. Outline cellulitis margin if present to monitor progression.

ALTERNATIVE — LOOP DRAIN TECHNIQUE

1. Make two small off-midline stab incisions across the abscess cavity (dependent and superior). Break loculations and irrigate.

2. Pass a soft vessel loop through one incision and out the other; tie loosely to maintain drainage. Cover with absorbent dressing.

3. Loop typically remains ~5–7 days, adjusted by drainage and comfort.

COMPLICATIONS / SIDE EFFECTS

1. Bleeding, pain flare, incomplete drainage/ recurrence; persistent sinus tract.

2. Cellulitis progression or systemic infection (rare after adequate drainage).

3. Scarring; rare neurovascular injury.

AFTERCARE & MONITORING

1. Daily showers or warm soaks; keep area clean and dry. Replace dressings when saturated.

2. Analgesia as needed. Avoid prolonged sitting and pressure on the cleft; consider a coccyx cushion.

3. Hair control: clip or depilate surrounding hair regularly after healing begins to reduce recurrence.

4. Antibiotics: consider if extensive cellulitis, systemic illness, immunocompromise, multiple lesions, or failure of I&D alone; choose per local guidance (e.g., MRSA coverage where appropriate).

5. Return if increasing pain, fever, spreading redness, persistent drainage >48–72 h, or if loop/packing dislodges early.

6. Plan surgical follow-up for consideration of definitive treatment once acute infection resolves.

DISPOSITION

1. Discharge with written instructions and recheck in 24–48 h if packed/looped, otherwise PRN.

2. Arrange referral to general/colorectal surgery for recurrent disease or poor response.

REFERENCES

NHS — Pilonidal sinus disease and abscess: overview and treatment. https://www.nhs.uk

American Society of Colon & Rectal Surgeons (ASCRS) — Patient information: Pilonidal Disease. https://fascrs.org

Healthdirect Australia — Pilonidal sinus. https://www.healthdirect.gov.au

MyHealth.Alberta.ca — Pilonidal cyst care instructions. https://myhealth.alberta.ca

Infectious Diseases Society of America (IDSA) — Skin & Soft Tissue Infection guidelines (open access) for antibiotic considerations. https://www.idsociety.org

GU & WOMEN'S HEALTH

BLADDER CATHETERIZATION — URETHRAL (MALE & FEMALE)

INDICATIONS

1. Acute urinary retention; chronic retention with complications (renal impairment, infection).
2. Need for accurate urine output monitoring in the acutely unwell.
3. Bladder irrigation/hematuria management; peri-operative use; protection of perineal wounds.
4. Palliative care comfort where appropriate.

CONTRAINDICATIONS / RED FLAGS (SEEK UROLOGY/ALTERNATIVE)

1. Suspected urethral injury (pelvic fracture, blood at meatus, gross hematuria, high-riding/non-palpable prostate).
2. Known urethral stricture, false passage, or recent urethral surgery (e.g., radical prostatectomy).
3. Severe resistance or pain on passage — **stop** and seek expert help.

4. Consider suprapubic catheter if long-term need with urethral contraindication.

CONSENT

5. Purpose: drain bladder, relieve retention, enable monitoring/irrigation.
6. Benefits: symptom relief, renal protection, accurate output.
7. Risks: infection (CAUTI), urethral trauma/ bleeding, false passage, paraphimosis (uncircumcised), discomfort, bladder spasm, autonomic dysreflexia (SCI).
8. Alternatives: intermittent catheterization, external (condom) catheter in males, trial without catheter (TWOC) if appropriate.

PREPARATION

1. Confirm indication; assess for red flags; check allergies (latex, chlorhexidine, lidocaine).
2. Explain procedure; privacy; chaperone as required; position: supine.
3. Hand hygiene; full sterile prep/drape; adequate lighting.
4. Preload 10 mL syringe with sterile water for balloon (verify catheter balloon size).
5. Consider topical anesthetic gel (e.g., 2% lidocaine jelly).

EQUIPMENT

1. Sterile catheterization kit: sterile gloves/drape, antiseptic swabs, lubricant/anesthetic gel, forceps, gauze.

2. Foley catheter (adult): **12–14 Fr female**, **14–18 Fr male** (start 14–16 Fr); **coude tip** if BPH/angulation.

3. Syringe with sterile water for balloon (commonly 10 mL; check catheter), closed drainage bag with hanger and securement device.

4. Optional: urine sample bottle for urinalysis/ culture prior to antibiotics.

PROCEDURE — MALE

1. Position supine; expose and prep glans/meatus; retract foreskin if present.

2. Clean from meatus outward. Grasp penis at 60–90° to torso to straighten urethra.

3. Instill **10–15 mL** anesthetic gel into urethra; wait 2–3 min.

4. Lubricate catheter; advance to the **Y-junction** (full length). Do **not** inflate balloon until urine flows.

5. If no urine (e.g., empty bladder), advance further to ensure intravesical position; then instill sterile saline to confirm free flow.

6. Inflate balloon with recommended volume (e.g., 10 mL sterile water). Gently withdraw until

resistance is felt at bladder neck.

7. Replace foreskin to prevent paraphimosis; connect closed bag and secure tubing.

PROCEDURE — FEMALE

1. Position supine, knees flexed/abducted; adequate lighting; separate labia with non-dominant hand (maintain cleanliness).

2. Clean urethral meatus anterior to vaginal introitus. If uncertain, a small amount of anesthetic gel can help identify meatus.

3. Lubricate catheter; insert **5–7 cm** until urine flows; advance another **2–3 cm** before balloon inflation.

4. Inflate balloon with recommended volume; gently withdraw to seat; connect and secure closed drainage.

IF DIFFICULTY / SPECIAL NOTES

1. Do **not** force against resistance. Try smaller size, additional lubrication, or **coude tip** (male).

2. If catheter enters vagina (female), **leave it in place** as a marker and use a new sterile catheter.

3. Consider intermittent catheterization if short-term decompression only.

4. For hematuria/clot retention, use **three-way

catheter** (16–22 Fr) for irrigation per local protocol.

COMPLICATIONS / SIDE EFFECTS

1. CAUTI, urethral trauma/bleeding, false passage, paraphimosis, bladder spasms, bypassing/ leakage, stones with long-term use.

2. Autonomic dysreflexia in spinal cord injury — monitor BP and manage promptly.

AFTERCARE & MONITORING

1. Secure catheter to thigh/abdomen; keep bag **below bladder**; maintain **closed system**; avoid kinks.

2. Perineal hygiene daily; empty bag using clean technique; avoid routine bladder washouts.

3. Review **ongoing need daily**; plan TWOC when possible; consider alternatives for long-term use.

4. Document size/type, balloon volume, batch/lot if available, urine characteristics/volume, and any complications.

DISPOSITION

1. Discharge with catheter care instructions if going home; arrange follow-up for TWOC/changes.

2. Urgent review for fever, lower abdominal pain, no drainage, gross hematuria/clots, or inability to flush if ordered.

REFERENCES

Centers for Disease Control and Prevention (CDC) — Guideline for Prevention of Catheter-Associated Urinary Tract Infections. https://www.cdc.gov

NICE CKS — Catheter-associated urinary tract infection: Prevention and management (open access). https://cks.nice.org.uk

NHS — Urinary catheter: overview and care. https://www.nhs.uk

Healthdirect Australia — Urinary catheter. https://www.healthdirect.gov.au

MyHealth.Alberta.ca — Indwelling urinary catheter care instructions. https://myhealth.alberta.ca

British Association of Urological Surgeons (BAUS) — Catheter care (patient information). https://www.baus.org.uk

BARTHOLIN GLAND ABSCESS — INCISION & DRAINAGE WITH WORD CATHETER

INDICATIONS

1. Fluctuant, painful labial mass consistent with Bartholin gland abscess.
2. Failure of conservative measures (analgesia, warm soaks) or systemic symptoms.
3. Recurrent cyst/abscess where fistulization tract formation is desired.

CONTRAINDICATIONS / CAUTIONS

1. Extensive cellulitis, systemic toxicity, or necrotizing infection — urgent surgical/ED assessment.
2. Atypical/solid mass, especially age >40 — consider malignancy; arrange gynecology review and biopsy as indicated.
3. Significant coagulopathy/anticoagulation (optimize and use meticulous hemostasis).
4. Latex allergy — use **latex-free** catheter/

balloon device.

CONSENT

1. Purpose: drain abscess and place Word catheter to create a short epithelialized tract to reduce recurrence.
2. Benefits: rapid pain relief, lower recurrence vs. simple I&D, office procedure.
3. Risks: pain, bleeding/hematoma, infection, catheter discomfort/expulsion, dyspareunia, recurrence; rare scarring or fistula.
4. Alternatives: simple I&D (higher recurrence), marsupialization, definitive surgery if recurrent.

PREPARATION

1. Assess for pregnancy and screen for STIs when risk factors present (take swabs/NAAT as per local guidance).
2. Analgesia/anesthesia: 1% lidocaine local infiltration; consider procedural sedation if needed.
3. Asepsis: cleanse vulva with chlorhexidine or povidone-iodine; drape. Position in lithotomy or frog-leg.
4. Antibiotics only if associated cellulitis/systemic features or STI risk; choose per local guidance.

EQUIPMENT

1. Word catheter (or small latex-free balloon catheter, e.g., 8–12 Fr if Word unavailable).
2. Scalpel (#11), curved hemostat, small scissors, forceps.
3. 10 mL syringe with 1% lidocaine; sterile saline for irrigation.
4. Gauze, swabs for culture/NAAT if indicated, sterile lubricant, adhesive dressing/pad.

PROCEDURE STEPS — OFF-MIDLINE I&D + WORD CATHETER

1. Identify mucosal surface at the inner aspect of the labia minora over the most fluctuant point, at ~4 or 8 o'clock position of the introitus (avoid midline).
2. Infiltrate with local anesthetic. Make a **~1–1.5 cm vertical mucosal incision** over the abscess; allow pus to drain. Collect swab if indicated.
3. Use a hemostat to gently explore and break loculations; irrigate the cavity with warm saline and remove debris/hair.
4. Insert the Word catheter tip into the abscess cavity. Inflate balloon with **2–3 mL sterile water** (adjust for comfort) and gently retract until balloon rests against the internal wall.
5. Seat the catheter with the stem lying within the introitus; trim if excessively long. Ensure

continued drainage.

6. Apply a pad; provide peri-care instructions.

COMPLICATIONS / SIDE EFFECTS

1. Bleeding, pain, secondary infection or cellulitis.

2. Catheter expulsion (especially in first 48 hours), discomfort during intercourse while in situ.

3. Recurrence despite catheter; rare fistula or scarring.

AFTERCARE & MONITORING

1. Warm sitz baths 1–2× daily after 24 hours; gentle hygiene; avoid intercourse/tampon use until comfortable.

2. Expect drainage for several days. Wear a sanitary pad. Analgesia as needed.

3. If catheter falls out within **<48 h**, attempt re-insertion; after several days and if asymptomatic, observation may be reasonable.

4. Leave catheter **in place ~2–4 weeks** to allow epithelial tract formation; arrange follow-up for review and removal if not expelled earlier.

5. Return precautions: fever, spreading redness, severe pain, persistent bleeding, inability to void.

DISPOSITION

1. Discharge with written instructions and follow-up in 1–2 weeks; additional visit at 2–4 weeks for

catheter removal if still in situ.

2. Plan STI counseling/testing as appropriate and discuss recurrence prevention.

REFERENCES

NICE CKS — Bartholin's cyst and abscess (open access). https://cks.nice.org.uk

NHS — Bartholin's cyst and abscess: overview and treatment. https://www.nhs.uk

RCOG — Patient information: Bartholin's cyst and abscess (open access leaflet). https://www.rcog.org.uk

Healthdirect Australia — Bartholin's cyst. https://www.healthdirect.gov.au

CDC — STI Treatment Guidelines (screening considerations). https://www.cdc.gov

PAP TEST — CERVICAL CYTOLOGY (SPECIMEN COLLECTION)

INDICATIONS

1. Cervical cancer screening per local program guidance.
2. Evaluation of abnormal bleeding or follow-up of prior abnormal screen (as directed by guidelines).

CONTRAINDICATIONS / CAUTIONS

1. Active, heavy bleeding that prevents adequate sampling (defer if possible).
2. Suspected pregnancy complications or placenta previa (do not proceed; refer).
3. Recent cervical surgery/biopsy: follow specialist advice; avoid endocervical brush in late pregnancy.
4. Active cervicitis: consider STI testing/ treatment; defer routine screening until treated if appropriate.

CONSENT

1. Purpose: collect cervical cells for cytology ± HPV testing.
2. Benefits: early detection of precancer/cancer.
3. Risks: brief discomfort, spotting, vasovagal symptoms; extremely rare infection.
4. Alternatives: per local guidance (primary HPV, co-testing, or interval screening).

PREPARATION

1. Explain steps; offer chaperone; confirm last menstrual period, contraception, pregnancy status, prior abnormal results.
2. Ask patient to avoid intercourse, vaginal medications/douching/tampons for **24–48 h** if feasible.
3. Have the patient empty bladder; position in lithotomy with adequate draping and lighting.

EQUIPMENT

1. Bivalve speculum (sizes: narrow/pediatric, medium, large); warm water for lubrication (avoid gel that may affect cytology).
2. Sampling device: broom-type (preferred single device) **or** Ayre spatula + endocervical brush (avoid brush in late pregnancy).
3. Liquid-based cytology (LBC) vial (e.g.,

PreservCyt/ThinPrep or SurePath) **or** glass slide + fixative if conventional smear used.

4. Labels/requisition with two identifiers, gloves, light source, cotton swabs (to clear excess mucus/blood from ectocervix).

PROCEDURE — SPECIMEN COLLECTION (LBC, BROOM-TYPE PREFERRED)

1. Insert warmed speculum gently; visualize cervix fully. Clear excess mucus with dry swab (avoid aggressive wiping).

2. Place broom with central bristles in os; rotate **5 full turns** maintaining contact with ecto- and endocervical epithelium.

3. Immediately rinse broom in LBC vial per manufacturer (e.g., swirl/press 10x); cap securely.

4. If using spatula + brush: rotate spatula **360°** around ectocervix; then insert endocervical brush **1–2 cm**, rotate **¼–½ turn** only, and rinse both in vial.

PROCEDURE — CONVENTIONAL SMEAR (IF LBC UNAVAILABLE)

1. Spread spatula sample **thinly and uniformly** on labeled slide **immediately**; fix within **10 seconds** to avoid air-drying.

2. Roll endocervical brush lightly on a second slide; fix immediately. Use appropriate spray/alcohol fixative.

SPECIMEN LABELING & REQUISITION

1. Label at bedside with **two identifiers**, date/time, and collector initials.

2. Requisition must include: patient identifiers, site (cervical/vaginal), pregnancy status/LMP, hysterectomy status, prior abnormal results, HPV request (if applicable), clinician info.

3. Note visible blood, inflammation, IUD, or unsatisfactory visualization.

SPECIAL SITUATIONS

1. Postmenopause/atrophy: smaller speculum; consider topical estrogen pre-treatment (per local program) if repeated insufficient samples.

2. Pregnancy: avoid endocervical brush in late pregnancy; use spatula or soft broom; stop if bleeding.

3. Adolescents/trauma history: smaller speculum, extra privacy and consent attention; consider pediatric speculum or side-wall retraction with swabs.

COMPLICATIONS / SIDE EFFECTS

1. Mild cramping/spotting, transient vasovagal symptoms.

2. Rare: significant bleeding or pain — stop and reassess.

AFTERCARE & FOLLOW-UP

1. Advise mild spotting may occur; avoid intravaginal products for 24 h if spotting.
2. Results communication plan: typical turnaround **1–3 weeks** (local).
3. Follow management per local guidelines (HPV triage, repeat interval, colposcopy referral). Provide safety-net for heavy bleeding, fever, severe pain.

DISPOSITION

1. Document device used, sample type (LBC vs smear), visualization adequacy, and any issues (bleeding, pain).
2. Ensure patient has contact method for results and understands next steps.

REFERENCES

BC Cancer — Cervix Screening: Pap Test Collection Guide (open access). https://www.bccancer.bc.ca

Alberta Health Services — Cervix Screening: Pap Test Collection (open access). https://screeningforlife.ca

Public Health England/NHS — Cervical screening: sample taker guidance (open access). https://www.gov.uk

World Health Organization — Cervical cancer screening and management resources (open access). https://www.who.int

Centers for Disease Control and Prevention (CDC) — Cervical cancer screening overview (open access). https://www.cdc.gov

www.ingramcontent.com/pod-product-compliance
Lightning Source LLC
Chambersburg PA
CBHW040922210326
41597CB00030B/5151